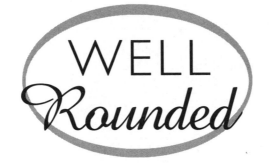

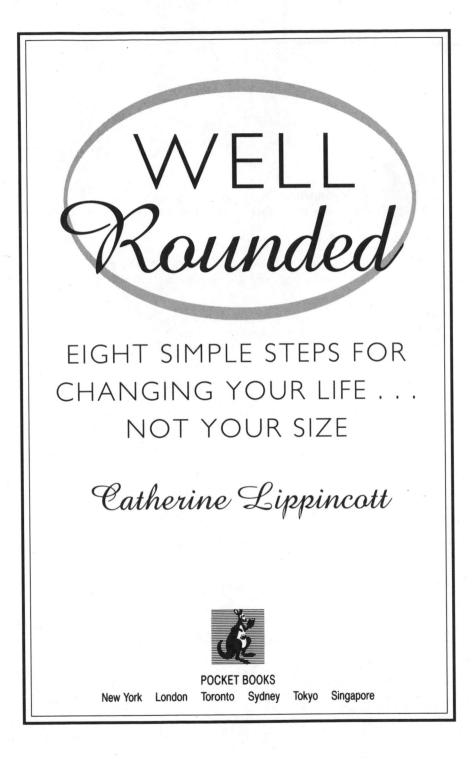

WELL
Rounded

EIGHT SIMPLE STEPS FOR CHANGING YOUR LIFE . . . NOT YOUR SIZE

Catherine Lippincott

POCKET BOOKS

New York   London   Toronto   Sydney   Tokyo   Singapore

POCKET BOOKS, a division of Simon & Schuster Inc.
1230 Avenue of the Americas, New York, NY 10020

Illustration of the body types for plus-size women from *Fashion Design for the Plus-Size* by Frances Leto Zangrillo, copyright © 1990 Fairchild Publications

Library of Congress Cataloging-in-Publication Data

Lippincott, Catherine.
    Well rounded : eight simple steps for changing your life . . . not your
size / Catherine Lippincott.
        p.   cm.
    Includes bibliographical references.
    ISBN: 0-671-54508-6
    1. Body image.   2. Overweight women—Psychology.   3.Obesity—
Psychological aspects.   4. Feminine beauty (Aesthetics)   5. Self-
esteem in women.   I. Title.
BF697.5.B63L56   1997
158'.1'082—DC20   96-41486
                                                            CIP

First Pocket Books hardcover printing January 1997

10   9   8   7   6   5   4   3   2   1

POCKET and colophon are registered trademarks of
Simon & Schuster Inc.

Text design by Stanley S. Drate/Folio Graphics Co. Inc.

Printed in the U.S.A.

"I dote on myself, there is that lot of me, and all so luscious."

—From "Song of Myself"
Walt Whitman

"A meaty woman, a healthy woman is so good looking. . . . It suggests a person who's not totally self-absorbed, who has other things to do."

—Fashion designer Isaac Mizrahi

"Deeply Dippy 'bout the curves you've got. . . . Deeply hot, hot for the curves you got."

—From the song "Deeply Dippy"
Right Said Fred

Contents

Contents

PART III

Leading the Way

Foreword

*W*hether you know it or not you have just taken the first step toward changing your life. Just the very fact that you have this book in your hands is an indication that you are on the path toward feeling better about yourself.

I know because I, too, am on the path. Changing your life is an ongoing process. We are never finished changing. Change keeps us young, healthy, and alive. And, contrary to what the media and society would have us believe, positive, lasting change happens from the *inside out*.

I write this for you as a large-size woman, a "woman of size." I am five feet, ten inches tall and wear a size 16. My current livelihood *depends* on my being a size 16. As a large-size model, I've noticed something happening over the past few years. Women of all shapes and sizes approach me on and off the runways of department stores around the country and tell me something very important.

Allow me to explain. Often stores hire me to be the "plus-size" model in an otherwise "regular-size" show. In other words, there will be eight "regular-size" models and me. After a show, as I am dressed in my street clothes and headed for my car, I am singled out time and time again by audience members who wait to talk to me. I couldn't believe it was happening at first. All my size 6 counterparts got dressed and walked out of the store without as much as a sideways glance from anyone. But women have something to say to me. They come up to me, look me straight in the eye, and say, "Thank you."

I am an average to good runway model, but I know they are not thanking me for my modeling prowess. They are thanking me for validating their bodies. They say how wonderful it makes them feel to see a "real person," a "real woman," a "woman whose body looks like mine" on the runway. Because I am one of the more than 40 million American women who wear over a size 12, I am part of their group, part of their reality. And, because of them, because of you, I have decided to write this book.

Being big isn't always easy. Over the years and through trial and error I have learned ways to change the way I look at myself, instead of changing the way I look. I have discovered how to live gracefully and meaningfully in my large-size body without anticipating life "when I lose weight." These changes took place *not* from a diet but rather from a conscious, gentle acceptance of my own body as it is. I will show you exactly how I got there and, by following the eight steps I outline, how you can get there too.

This is *not* another diet book or exercise regimen. It *is* a source for you to improve the quality of your life; an inside-and-out, self-awareness and fashion test ground complete with the tools necessary to help you live your life to the fullest each and every day. I'll show you how to make immediate and noticeable changes. I promise instant results. You will look and feel great TODAY, not tomorrow, in six weeks, or a year from now.

This is for you. Onward!

Part One

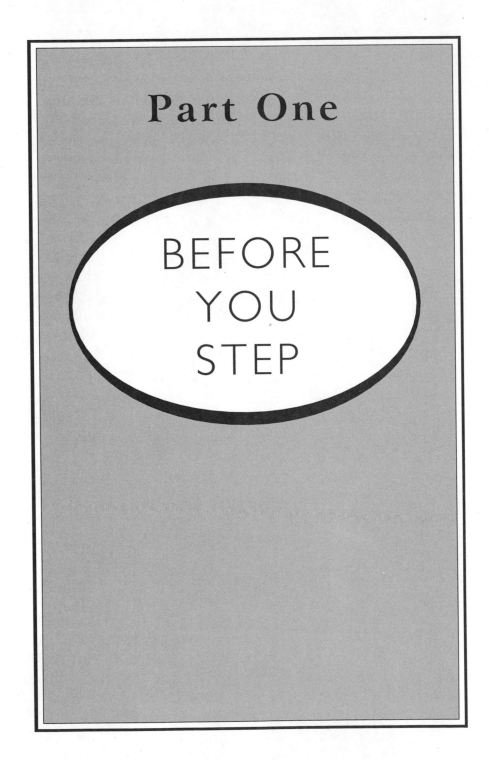

BEFORE
YOU
STEP

*I*f you are "rounded"—you know, large, big, heavy, shapely, Rubenesque, zaftig, or curvy, size 12 to 28 or 30, or 40 or 50—I know how you feel right now. I know because I am big and I have felt the same way too.

I understand those feelings of desperation, helplessness, and hopelessness associated with weight. I know the feeling that everyone else is "thin" and "in" on life, loving, living, laughing . . . and the feeling that we are excluded from that happiness by virtue of our size. It's as if there's this very desirable "thin club" and as hard as we try to starve, exercise, and diet our way into the club, we can't seem to get our hands on a membership card. And, if we ever do, it's only fleeting and vanishes the minute the pounds inevitably creep back on. They say membership has its privileges, but I've never seen them. The one time I think I *might* have qualified as a member, I was too weak from dieting to know or care that I was in the club.

I know the sense of impending doom of habitually "going on a diet." It is a sadness in the heart that can barely be described in words. I remember feeling like I was losing my best friend. I could never sleep the night before I was going to begin a new diet. I would awake numerous times during the night and go down to the kitchen for repeated "last meal" rituals—last good-byes to my best friend. Just one more cookie, one last taste of bread and butter, a final scoop of ice cream. I had to say

3

good-bye to all my old friends and it was always very, very sad. In mourning, I cried before each "diet" began.

And then there's the feeling of extreme deprivation from "being on a diet" because you are in a perpetual state of self-induced punishment. The only thing that made me feel better about being on a diet was the fact that I had an automatic rebuttal for insulting remarks or comments about my weight. "Yes, but I *am* on a diet now." As if I were in the process of fixing something . . . something that I later learned was never broken to begin with.

And how about that guilty/happy/embarrassed/satiated feeling you get when you "cheat" on a diet? It feels so good to eat and to justify every mouthful with the promise "I'll start tomorrow for *real*." And, as we all know, tomorrow never comes.

And these feelings are elementary compared to the rock-bottom despair we feel as we regain all the weight we just worked so hard to lose. That has to be the worst of all. I recall being eighteen years old and losing control of my eating after a five-month medically supervised fast. I had been bingeing uncontrollably for weeks, and the weight was reappearing at a alarmingly rapid rate. I remember being in my bedroom sobbing uncontrollably, rocking back and forth and talking to myself out loud to try to calm myself down. I kept repeating the words, "It hurts. It hurts. It hurts so much." The shame and guilt we feel from regaining weight does hurt. In fact, dieting itself hurts. It hurts because we are punishing ourselves for a "crime" that does not deserve punishment. The repeated hurt from weight regain hurts so much that it can permanently damage our soul, our self-worth, our very being.

I know the feeling of being called names out loud on

the street, whispered in dressing rooms, not-so-silently snickered by kids on the bus, and, most devastating of all, names called to our faces, in our own homes, by our own family and friends who are trying to "help" us.

I also know all too well the feelings you might be having of not wanting to get dressed because everything you really want to wear is tight, uncomfortable, hot, itchy, cutting, binding, and obtrusive. And I know how hard it is to find clothing that fits and is comfortable at the same time—meaning it won't show rolls, will keep you cool, and doesn't let your legs rub together.

These are all feelings I know firsthand. I have had them all and then some. For many years, I lived my life with these feelings and in search of a way to become thin, so all these feelings would disappear. And it never happened that way . . . until.

It never changed until I decided to stop punishing myself for my size and start figuring out ways to live happily and productively inside the body I have. Ever since I made that shift in perception, that change in attitude, I have embraced and celebrated the well-rounded me. I gave up dieting, and gave in to nurturing, loving, and celebrating the body I have. The eight steps in this book will walk you through the process of nurturing, loving, and celebrating your own body

This is *not* a diet book. You will *not* find an eight-step diet regimen to follow. There will be no calorie or fat gram charts. I have had enough of those, haven't you? In fact, I have bookshelves lined with them. Starting with the "Jean Nidetch Story" (Ms. Weight Watchers herself) working through Dr. Stillman's water diet, Dr. Atkins's low-carbos diet and on into the Scarsdale, the Beverly Hills, the Pritikin, the Royal Canadian Air Force, and the Cambridge diets.

This book is a success story, but a success story of a different kind. It is not an "I-was-fat-and-miserable-but-now-I'm-thin-and-happy" story. Those tales never meant anything to me. Who cares if someone lost fifty pounds and as a result claims that she got a fabulous job, met Prince Charming, or acquired more money than the sultan of Brunei? I never believed that those stories were real. Did you? And, as we all know from statistics, over 90 percent of those people who lose weight on a diet gain it all back again. This is a real success story. It will have a happy ending. It is the story of how you learn to live gracefully and lovingly inside the body you have.

My Success

The success story that I have to tell is how I learned to live my real life, gracefully and fully, inside my real body—regardless of a number on a scale or a size in a dress. I base my success on knowing that sometimes I have a bad day, and sometimes I have a great one. Sometimes I wake up "heavier" and sometimes "lighter." Some days everything drives me crazy and other days are effortlessly joyful. I have found my success in being able to accept and embrace both sides of every coin.

For so long, I believed that I was having a bad day or a bad moment or a bad relationship or a bad job because I was fat. *Not* true. Bad things do not happen to people based on a dress size. Life just doesn't work that way.

I am a whole woman as I am today, whatever I might weigh, and so are you. I am whole because I love and approve of myself no matter what the number on the scale says. I love and approve of you no matter what you weigh. And through these pages, you will learn to love and approve of yourself and the body you have.

My Body

Are you curious about my body? I'm curious about yours. Maybe you'll send me a picture of you and let me know if you like what you've read in these pages. I am constantly fascinated with bodies. Each is so different, so unique, so beautiful in its own way. Some years back I worked in a well-known, upscale, plus-sized women's store and was constantly amazed by the variety of body types and shapes. There is so much variation. I helped dress hundreds of women, and no two were alike. Two women may both wear a size 22, but I can guarantee you that their bodies are radically different from one another.

Me? I've got curves and bumps and muscles and flesh. Hips, breasts, thighs, and belly. They are all part of my beautiful body. It is as unique as I am.

I am five feet, ten inches tall and weigh somewhere between 210 and 220 pounds. I can't give you an exact weight, because it changes all the time. I've come to realize that we are never *one* weight or *one* dress size. We are constantly changing. But more on that later. Let's talk about you. Let me get to know you. Are you a lot like I am?

Who Are You?

Have you ever told yourself you will be happy if you lose five (or fifty) pounds? Have you ever bought an item of clothing that is a size too small, thinking you will lose weight to fit into it? Have you ever thought that you couldn't go to a party, a wedding, or a special event because of the way you look or feel?

You and I both have, at some point in our lives, answered yes to these questions. We have allowed our weight, and the negative feelings associated with our weight, to delay or deny us the pleasure of living fully and happily. Maybe we passed up an opportunity for a new relationship. Maybe it was a new job or a promotion. Maybe it was just a change to get out and have some fun—all because we believed we should postpone our lives until we reached some magic, special number on the scale. And until that moment we were not going to allow ourselves to participate in any of life's wonderful and exciting activities.

Marcia Millman, in her book *Such a Pretty Face*, describes the phenomenon of postponing one's life:

> Because her unacceptable body comes to stand in her mind for everything wrong in her life, she also imagines that being fat is the cause of all her troubles. Her response is to cease living in the present. Instead, she turns all her thoughts and attentions to the future when she shall be slender. Her present life circumstances are discounted as temporary, preparatory, not the real thing. Real life, she reasons, will start after she loses weight. The belief in a "before-and-after" transformation is a towering and universal fantasy.

Postponing

The universal fantasy. Our lives will be complete when we are thin. We postpone, deny, and delay until we weigh less. We make excuses. Excuses to others, but mostly excuses to ourselves. I was constantly making excuses for myself.

I would reason with myself about why my life wasn't perfect, and blame it on my weight. I was absolutely positive that I would never have a boyfriend until I got "thin." I thought that if I bought clothes in a smaller size I would automatically be motivated to lose weight to fit into them. And how many times have I had every intention of going to the party, but in the final hour decided I didn't feel good and stayed home instead, victimized by weight and a slave to size?

Blaming weight for everything is easy to do. Excuses were my guards who protected me from the outside world as well as from accepting, loving, and celebrating myself—myself at any weight, any size. Me . . . Catherine . . . a wonderful person worth loving, fat or thin, or anywhere in between.

My Genetic Bigness

I am the thirty-two-year-old daughter of a long line of large, healthy women. I knew and loved my maternal great-grandmother, Gram, only when I was very young. She was in her late nineties when I was a little girl. I remember visiting her in the big house with the three big porches in Virginia. She slept in a big bed. She had a big lap . . . a comfortable lap, and a comfortable, big laugh to go along with it. She had a big box of ginger snaps, which she would share with her great-grandchildren after we took our vitamins. The *big* I remember about her was always a *good* big.

My grandmother Mimi was glamorous with a capital

G. She had seven marriage proposals, and chose my grandfather because "he had nice hands." I always thought my grandparents were the most dashing couple. Mimi was five feet, eight inches, considered tall for a woman of her era, and always wore a size 14 or 16. When I think more carefully about her body, I recall that she had a tummy. She used to joke about it. She'd say it was as big as a watermelon. We would laugh, I would pat it and tell her that it wasn't so big, and then we would go downstairs and enjoy a delicious lunch together.

Now as an adult, remembering that Mimi had a tummy, acknowledging the fact, the realness of it, the roundness of it, has had great impact on my recent journey into body awareness. She had a female's typical *rounded belly* and everyone still thought she was the most wonderful, beautiful woman ever. Could it be possible that I could love myself *and* my own fleshy, rounded lower abdomen? Or even that others would love me *and* my curves below the belt?

My mother has battled her weight all her life. Never "obese," she was encouraged by her mother (Mimi) to adhere to the fifties ideal of beauty—the perfect circle-skirted, sweater-set and pearled, bright-eyed, marriage-minded size 8. She was sent to a famous "reducing spa" when she was only sixteen years old. Her weight fluctuated all her early life and she got married as a big-boned but acceptable size 12.

I am the product of a big family . . . mostly big women. Did you know that if just one of your parents is "big," you stand a 40 percent chance of being "big" yourself? And if *both* of your parents are big, there is an 80 percent chance that you too will carry more weight. Basically, our tendency to be larger is inherited. At 9 lbs, 2 ounces, I was born with the 80 percent chance that I would grow up to be a well-rounded woman of size. I don't know why this came as such a shock to my family, but it did. Maybe it has something to do with being born in Texas.

What can I say about Texas? It's the land where everything is supposed to be big . . . except the women. In Texas, you are encouraged to have big cars, big houses, big hair, and big appetites. Remember the saying, "Everything is *big* in Texas"? I came to learn early that women are the one glaring exception to the "big" rule. In fact, Texans like their women rather petite. Maybe it's because they decided that *something* had to remain small so as to make everything else look BIG by comparison. Keep your cattle big, but your little gal small.

Maybe it was the era, or maybe it was the state; either way, my family was a little shocked when I was the biggest kindergartner. And increasingly alarmed when I was the fleshiest first grader, having to have my school uniforms altered so that they would fit my chubby seven-year old body. And with this, my diet history begins. I bet you have one too. Does it sound anything like this?

Profile of a Dieter

I am a little girl in the first grade. A close family member thinks I should lose weight. He makes a deal with me, whereby he will pay me 75 cents a week for adhering to a diet he found printed on the back of a cereal box. I comply for a couple of weeks, not really wanting the money, but rather his approval and love. Yes, I lost weight. Yes, I regained it—plus some.

I am eleven years old. I am now in the fifth grade and I love my reading and writing classes. I worry at the

11

start of each new school year because the gym uniforms don't have elastic waists and I am already in the biggest size. Mom decides it is time for me to go to the local, well-known "diet doctor." Looking back, and as far as I can make out, a diet doctor is a real, live M.D. who has no compunction about diagnosing a fake thyroid condition so that he may prescribe low-grade "speed" pills to induce weight loss. My mother swears by this man and his pills because they got her thin again after she had my baby brother. I start to take the pills, not even knowing what a thyroid is. I tell my mom that they make me dizzy and that they make my heart race and flutter. She says that it means they are working and that I will be losing weight soon. I comply because I know she'll love me more if I am thinner. Yes, I lost weight. Yes, I regained it—plus some.

I am fourteen years old and entering the eighth grade. I have to miss the school pep rallies on Friday afternoons because Fridays are the weight hypnotist days. Mom and I go together. We are led into a darkened room (lecture hall style) with about thirty other people (mostly women in their forties). Dr. G. comes out of a side door and leads a relaxation session, telling our subconscious minds that we will not feel hunger or want food. Although my instincts tell me that feeling hunger and wanting food are natural human needs, I figure that he must know best and I try hard to be hypnotized into thinness. Yes, I lost weight. Yes, I regained it—plus some.

I am seventeen years old, entering my senior year of high school. My dad takes me out to dinner (a steak restaurant) and tells me point blank that *No one will ever love me unless I lose weight.* And that he has the solution. A new weight-loss "cure" whereby I give up solid foods and begin a medically supervised "fast" with the aid of a powder-and-water mixture. Presumably, I will continue this fast for months or at least until I get thin enough so that *someone* will love me.

He tells me that Larry Hagman of *Dallas* and *I Dream of Jeannie* fame has had great success on this program. I fast for five months. I lose 120 pounds—along with some patches of my hair and my balance. In the fourth and fifth months of the fast, I generally wake up in the morning, get out of bed, and immediately black out. I wonder if Larry Hagman faints too. I get used to this, though, because I know my family is very proud of me. Yes, I lost weight. Yes, I regained it—all of it—plus some.

I am nineteen years old and just finishing my sophomore year of college. I now hate myself and the way my body looks so much that I join the ranks and legions of family members who are grasping for weight-loss solutions for me. I check myself into a fancy, two-month weight-loss clinic in Durham, North Carolina. All I really remember is that everything is weighed and measured every day. You. Your food. Your sweat. Your pee. "Behavior modification" is the buzz phrase that accesses you to group therapy (a group of hungry, well-rounded people sitting around talking about McRib sandwiches). During my stint at the clinic, there is a well-known, chronically "overweight" actor in our group. He has been there several months already and provided some much-needed humor. Unfortunately, he is kicked out of the program prematurely and sent home as a punishment for slipping salt tablets into everyone's urine samples on a particularly gloomy day. Yes, I lost weight. Yes, I regained it—plus some.

This is only a partial sampling of the dieting attempts I made between the ages of six and twenty-five.

The diet mentality ruled my life during those years. During that time I would have described my life in terms of (a) the diet I was currently on, (b) the diet that had just failed, (c) or the new diet that I was about to try. I lost and regained hundreds of pounds. Yo-yoing became part of my life. I dragged through days, weeks, months, and years, looking forward to a life in the future when I would be thin. My family equated thinness with happiness and tried to help me find my way to the mecca of thinness. Do I blame my family for trying to help me lose weight? Absolutely not. They love me and were trying to do what they felt was best for me. Do I blame society and the media for convincing my family (and the world) that thin equals happy? Yes.

Where Are Our Bigger, Better Role Models?

I loved Barbie dolls with all their plastic, unrealistic curves. I think I recognized early on that she was someone I could never be. What I didn't realize was that she was someone that *no woman* could ever be by natural means. How may women do you know with such small feet and hands? No hips, huge bosom, and tiny waist? I believe Barbara (as she would probably want to be addressed today) was a harbinger of the unrealistic, photo-retouched "ideal" body images we see gracing the fashion magazines today.

Growing up, I wanted to be either a ballet dancer or an airline stewardess. Talk about setting myself up for disappointment—but in the 1960s in Texas, ballet dancers and stewardesses were the working-women role models of the day, as the female "power exec" had not yet surfaced. I didn't have a "traditional" ballet dancer's body and stewardesses had weight restrictions, so both seemed fairly unobtainable as a young girl. I had no role models in sight anywhere—especially ones that might have a non-Twiggy body.

So, I looked to television for an answer. In the 1970's, Bill Cosby's *The Fat Albert Show* was one of my favorite Saturday morning cartoons. I would watch this show alone without my little brother or friends around. I feared they would make fun of me . . . a fat kid watching Fat Albert would draw too close a parallel and open myself up for immediate ridicule. I continued to struggle in finding someone—anyone—to relate to in terms of my body.

Jim Henson's Miss Piggy became popular when I was about fourteen or fifteen. I recall buying the Miss Piggy Pin-Up Calendar. She (Piggy) was curvy, and confident—always getting what she wanted (with the exception of Kermit the Frog) and looking very glamorous in the process. My intrigue with her came crashing to a halt the day a family member saw the calendar hanging in my bedroom, and was disgusted at my apparent "connection" with a talking pig who wore a feather boa. "She's a *pig*. People are making *fun* of her, Catherine. Don't you understand?" All I understood was that she was secure with a body that didn't look anything like Barbie's but much more like mine.

Things have not improved a great deal today. We are still in need of more positive role models who live and love inside their well-rounded bodies. There is, however, one place to turn for constant support and reinforcement: Art. Specifically, paintings and sculpture that depict the female form as it exists—fleshy, rounded, full, and beautiful beyond words.

Bodies like ours are represented everywhere. All we need to do is to look beyond the magazine rack and the television. *Our* bodies are in the Louvre and the Prado and the Metropolitan Museum of Art. The Uffizzi, the Hermitage, the National Gallery, and the Cairo Museum. *Our* curves are carved in marble, stone, and alabaster and shaped by the hands and brush strokes of geniuses.

Twentieth-century fashion photographers do not set the perimeters for *our* bodies. We have been immortalized by Michelangelo, Botticelli, Rubens, and Renoir. These artists modeled their goddesses after *our* fleshy, round, strong curves.

One doesn't have to look far to find classical inspiration. Sitting in the Library of Congress my gaze turns upward to the ceiling of the rotunda in the main reading room. Eleven-foot statues encircle the ceiling—each a female form representing the eight characteristic features of civilized life and thought. Made of gleaming white plaster, ideals such as *commerce, religion, philosophy*, and *poetry* are personified by the female form. These are not small ideals . . . and these are not small women. Their voluptuous bodies represent beauty and strength. I see generous hips and ample arms, rounded bellies, strong, sturdy legs, and full waists. You or I could have been the life models for these statues. A model from the pages of a current fashion magazine would have been laughed out of the sculptor's studio.

Our bodies are the bodies that have been idealized and envied for ages. Our bodies represent health, wealth, and classical beauty known from the Greek and Roman goddesses. How that concept has been lost in our time I do not know.

We Need a Map

So, here we are now. Today. As I sit writing these words I am wearing a size 16. Some days my size 16 skirts are tighter, some days they are looser. Sound familiar? Weight is still an issue in my life. It always will be. What has changed my life is *how I perceive my weight*. Part of this process of looking at my weight in a new light led me to the conclusion that we, who compose over one third of the female population, have had no guidelines or standards to follow when it comes to looking or feeling good about ourselves. We have no road map, no directions, no signs or signals to follow.

In fact, the only direction we *have* been given, loudly and clearly and repeatedly, from the outside world is to *lose weight*. Period. End of discussion. "Stop eating. Go on a diet. That's how you'll solve your problems, succeed at work, have a better relationship."

In general, women of size have been excluded in all facets of their lives. Because it is more fashionable these days to be slim, we have been denied access to the information and products that could potentially enhance and enrich our lives. And nowhere is this more evident than in the lack of information on:

How to balance the external messages we receive that tell us how our bodies "should" look. We are bombarded with unrealistic images of women without being given the information on how to relate them to our lives.

How to believe in our own worth, no matter what size we wear. We are led to believe that we are somehow not up to par because of our size.

How to relax—taking the essential time to repair and rejuvenate ourselves daily. It is generally believed that women of size are relaxing too much (are lazy), and that this is part of our weight "problem."

How to relate to our bodies, sustaining a healthy, hands-on, attentive relationship with the body we have. Society and the media lead us to believe that we don't deserve a relationship with our body unless (or until) it is "thin."

How to assess our positives—making a personalized inventory of everything we like about ourselves, both inside and out.

How to dress and accessorize with confidence and style. We are told it doesn't matter what we wear or how we wear it until we are thinner. We are instructed to dress to look "thin," not how to look attractive, stylish, or appropriate.

How to relate to food. The information we are given is to diet and deny ourselves food, rather than to reassess how we relate to our food.

How to move. We are warned that exercise can be too difficult and dangerous for women of size. We have been taught only that movement is related to weight loss rather than to a general sense of well-being.

Simple Steps for Changing Your Life, Not Your Size

What I came to realize was that neither society nor the media offers us the positive reinforcement or the accepting and supportive advice we need. As a result, I made it my personal goal to create a special set of guidelines or steps to follow, tailored just for well-rounded women. This is a road map, some signs, a few suggestions . . . concise, simple steps that have worked for me in improving the way I look and feel. And the amazing thing is that the *only* thing you have to change is the *way you think about yourself.*

I am not a doctor or a psychologist or a nutritionist. I am a woman who decided to create her own set of guidelines for living well in my generously shaped body. I wasn't getting the information I needed from my family, my doctor, TV talk shows, *Vogue* or *Cosmopolitan.* So I made up my own rules. Some of them are common sense and some I have discovered through trial and error. Part II of this book will walk you through each of the eight steps for changing your life, not your size. I created the steps out of my own need, and they have helped me dramatically change my life and the way I feel about my body. I feel confident they will do the same for you.

Tools

In order to get to work and begin to initiate positive change, we need the proper tools to work with. I will give you these tools. At the end of each step you will find what I call the "Toolbox." The Toolbox is your own personal working record and analysis of aspects of yourself and your life. It is designed to be interactive. That means you are encouraged to fill out the questions and fill in the blanks, take notes, and scribble thoughts. The Toolbox holds the tools you will need to relearn successfully the process of loving yourself every day.

Some activities you find in the Toolbox will be

straightforward and simple, to drive home a straightforward but simple and important point. Some of the activities will require thought and reflection. They will request that you examine parts of yourself closely, maybe even parts you forgot were there.

Don't feel that you have to race through and complete the Toolbox at the end of each step. There are issues and ideas presented that might stir up old emotions. You might cry. You might laugh. I hope you do both. I certainly did while I was writing them. You may want to skip certain Toolbox activities and jump ahead to another. There is no certain order in which you should complete the activities. I do hope, however, that you will make an effort to complete each and every one of the activities in your own time and in your own way. The steps hold vital information and it is by working through the Toolbox exercises at the end of each step that your own change begins.

How It Works

When do I start feeling better? How long does it take? Will I lose weight? How do the steps work? These are all very good questions. Let's take them one at a time.

When will I begin to feel better about myself? Immediately. I have designed this book to help you initiate immediate positive change. By completing the Toolbox activities, you will recognize and rediscover long-forgotten attributes. You will feel better about yourself no matter what the scale says. Today. Now. Not tomorrow or next week.

How long will it take? To change your life successfully and continue to feel better and better about yourself as a well-rounded woman will take the rest of your life, I hope. This is a process, a journey. And we are always traveling, moving, and learning . . . changing, loving, and growing.

Will I lose weight? In this ongoing process, weight loss may be a by-product of your newfound self-esteem. In other words, not until you realize and recognize how wonderful you are right now will you be able to change anything about your life. Including your weight.

How do the Steps work? Part II is where you'll find the eight steps for changing your life, not your size. Some of the steps may be easier than others. Remember, changing your life is a process. You may not be able to complete them all on first reading. In fact, I hope you will read through this book once, and then return to the parts you found challenging and work through them one by one. The steps are as varied in nature as any one day in your life could be. Some steps will ask you to tackle clearing the clutter from your closets. Others will ask you to make time each day to think and reflect. The idea is that we must dabble a little in each area, every day, to stimulate the process of change.

This process is not a one-time, one-shot deal. This is the beginning of a process, of many processes. We will be changing the way we think about our bodies. That, in and of itself, is an enormous task. The way we perceive ourselves is ingrained at an early age and old thought patterns are stubborn and sometimes resistant to change. And because of the challenging nature of this process, I want to begin by arming you with a strong and powerful tool. Your team.

Teams

No one wants to face the world alone. We perform at our optimal level when surrounded and encouraged by the emotional support of others. Teams. Team management. Team sports. People who can pick up the ball if you drop it. People who know when to say, "You're tired, let me carry the ball for a while." People who boost you up, not bring you down. People who know when to give a word or two of advice and when not to. People who like you today, liked you yesterday, and you know will still like you tomorrow. People who have the ability to see some special part of you. These are the people who will make up your own personal team—your own collective force of positive energy and acceptance.

If you are wondering who they are and how you might go about finding them, let me start by saying that one has already found you. I may not be able to be with each of you face-to-face, but I'd like you to consider me as part of your team. We have been brought together through these pages for whatever reason and through whatever circumstances. I want to be your first team member—or at least a cheerleader!

Teams can be small or large. They can start small and grow larger, or reduce in size over time. They can be family members, friends, work associates, or the lady you talk to at the bus stop. They have to be people who make you feel great about yourself, who celebrate you for what you are; not what you weigh. Let me share a few of my team members with you so that you'll get the idea:

BERTHA: Our family's housekeeper and baby-sitter for the past forty years. She has been an inspiration and stalwart of support and unconditional love.

PUSHA: Part of my "beauty team," she does my manicures and pedicures. She has watched my life change and grow over the past eight years and has provided love, support, and insight—not to mention the most beautiful nails in town!

DENISE: My fitness specialist and my very first aerobics teacher. She is a New York-based personal trainer who has known and worked diligently and lovingly with my body in its many different shapes and sizes.

MALISSA: My best girlfriend. We lived down the hall from each other in college, and since we met fourteen years ago, we have weathered multiple life changes— including body changes, relationship changes, career changes, city changes, and just about every other change you can imagine—together. Throughout the ups and downs we support each other unconditionally.

LYNNE: Lynne is my nutritionist and a top expert on food issues. She is an extensive source of facts and data about eating, weight, and food and taught me how to live comfortably and reasonably within a body that isn't "thin." She does not believe in deprivation or dieting.

JOY AND BART: Owners of The Candle Café, a health-conscious restaurant in New York City. They are healers, believers, and motivators. They feed my body and my soul.

BILLY B.: A world-famous makeup artist whom I have known for more than ten years. He believes that true beauty comes from the inside and he makes others feel beautiful just being around him. Billy has loved and supported me through many weight ups and downs.

See? It's a mixed bag of people who love and accept me and always have. As I look at the partial list, I realize that none of the above-mentioned team members even live in the same city where I now live! But I know they are with me, no matter what. Just identifying your team will make you feel stronger. Even if it is only one person. You will know that you have backup support whenever you need it.

Onward!

I've been a size 24 and I once was a size 12 for about six hours, I think. I remain a little unsure about it because it was at the end of a "medically supervised" five-month fast and during those months I didn't have enough energy to read the label in a dress. (If you have been on one of these medically supervised fasts, you'll know what I mean.) These days, however, my body is arranged at a comfortable size 16—which for me is a very realistic and happy medium.

It took awhile, and although I still work on these issues daily, I have learned to stop basing my worth on my weight. Within these steps I will show you how to stop making excuses and begin to enjoy your own life *today*, not next week, next year, or after the next diet. You will look and feel better immediately. There will be no need for a "next diet" ever again.

This book is not meant to be used as an excuse to "stay fat," or to "stay thin," or to "stay" anything at all. It's about feeling better as you are now, and watching the positive fallout reverberate through all areas of your life. Together we will be working toward the goal of self-acceptance and self-love, which supersede and overrule any diet. From here on out, your "diet" will consist of everything you choose to create self-awareness, enhance self-acceptance, and heighten your well-being, physically and mentally and spiritually.

It *is* possible to be everything you want to be and do

everything you want to do right now. The key is to stop making weight your excuse. Actually, the great news is that you are only one page away from changing your life forever—learning to nurture, love, and celebrate the body you have.

Part Two

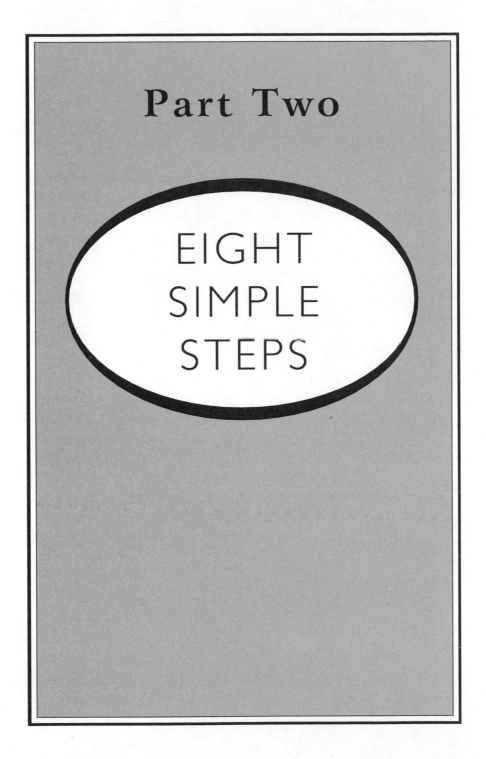

EIGHT
SIMPLE
STEPS

*O*nly eight of them. No more. No less. Simple because they are straightforward and easy to understand. I am a real "bottom line" type of person. I like to be given the necessary information and then begin putting it to work. True to form, this book is a bottom line book. There is no extraneous material floating around for you to have to muddle through. After reading and working through the eight steps, you will notice immediate changes in the way you look and feel about yourself. I created these steps to be a road map . . . guidelines and techniques to help you live joyfully and gracefully inside the body you have.

I suggest, the first time, that you read the eight steps in order. Then you can go back and re-read or work on any one (or several) of your choice. Try to complete as many of the Toolbox exercises (found at the end of each step) as you can. These are "practice fields" in which you are able to explore each step further, applying the concepts to your own life and needs.

Like a smile, a good feeling or a happy thought, the eight steps start from deep *inside* you and work their way outward. Change begins on the very next page with Step 1.

*T*here is an Indian
proverb or axiom that says
that everyone is a house
with four rooms, a physical, a
mental, an emotional and a
spiritual. Most of us tend to live in
one room most of the time but,
unless we go into every room
every day, even if only to
keep it aired, we are not a
complete person.

—RUMER GODDEN

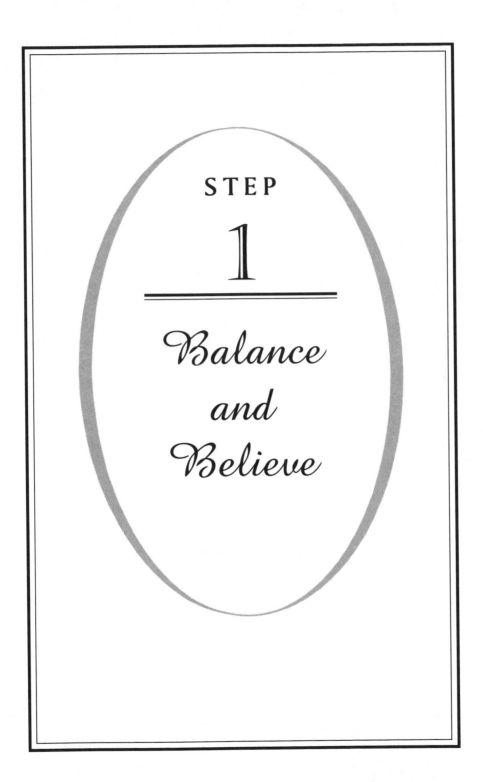

STEP

1

Balance
and
Believe

*W*e begin the process of changing your life by making subtle but essential changes in the way you perceive the body you have. I want you to embrace a new outlook and embark on a slow but steady change in attitude. In Step 1, I won't be asking you to do anything more than consider the way you have been approaching your body and your life inside that body.

The two cornerstones of a new, well-rounded you are your ability to *balance*—keeping your expectations in check and expertly juggling different areas of your life each day, and to *believe*—trusting in your instincts and the power you have to love and accept yourself as you are today. Creating a *balance* in your life and *believing* that you can live gracefully inside the body you have are the new thought patterns you will use to begin changing your life.

From the start, I want you to adopt a new way of thinking and make the small yet highly significant moves in your own mind from victimized to *victorious*, from insecure to *confident*, and from scattered to *serene*. I encourage you to recognize and celebrate the joyously satisfied, well-rounded woman you have the potential to be. In order to do this, you need to *balance* your life and *believe* in your worth.

Balance

Years of yo-yo dieting and weight obsession have caused women of size to swing far off kilter in the way we perceive our bodies. Fixations about food, compulsive dieting, and overexercising have all contributed to an unbalanced perspective with a primarily negative slant.

Restoring *balance* in your life is essential to repairing your self-image, especially where your body is concerned. Balance means that you are willing to release those old "all or nothing," "good food / bad food," "fat or thin," "feast or fast" attitudes and replace them with an innate understanding of how your body works, combined with newfound respect and forgiveness. Establishing a body-positive balance begins once you understand three simple concepts.

1. BALANCE YOUR PERCEPTION OF BEAUTY: HEALTHY, BEAUTIFUL BODIES COME IN ALL SHAPES AND SIZES.

There is a balance between hundreds upon thousands upon millions of body types in the world. Each one is uniquely different from the next. In learning how to balance the body we have in the landscape of the world, it is important to recognize and acknowledge that we can be healthy, beautiful, strong . . . and big. And it might be big in any number of different ways. Big and tall. Big and round. Big and strong. Big and soft. Big and lean. Big and sexy. Big and short. Big and big.

The best way to understand this concept is to sharpen your observation skills by sitting somewhere and watching bodies go by. You can do it anywhere; in your own front yard, in a mall, at the grocery store, in the line for the car pool, or at a restaurant. Learn to be expert at watching bodies. Begin to notice them all, and everything about them. Notice the shape, the size, and the form. Some are big, some are small. Some women have big frames—large bones, wide shoulders—some have smaller features and shorter limbs. There are lean bodies, leggy bodies, full bodies, meaty bodies, top heavy, bottom heavy, middle heavy, and all-over heavy bodies. Muscular, thick, dense frames or bodies that look like they could blow away in the wind. Tall or petite? [Did you know that in the fashion industry, the word "petite" refers *only* to height? "Petite" means five feet, five inches or shorter. The word has nothing to do with weight, body size or shape, *only* height. A woman can be petite and weight 100, 200, or 300 pounds. It only means that she is not taller than five feet, five inches.]

As you are watching bodies go by, start to look even closer, picking out distinguishing body features. Notice which features or characteristics you see first. More than likely, your eye will travel to the bodies or body parts that are noticeably different from the images we see in fashion magazines. Your natural tendency will be to criticize first. That's okay. It's only natural. We are bombarded daily with unrealistic images of women and instructed to attempt to look just like them. Concentrate on looking past the magazine stereotypes, and begin to single out beautiful features from every body you see. Train your eye to find a shapely calf, seek out a perfect "pear shape," notice a feminine bustline and cleavage, admire strong, square shoulders or well-proportioned, rounded hips. Look at each body in a new way, and challenge yourself to discover the unique, inherent, and individual beauty each body has to offer.

Each of our bodies has something beautiful and wonderful about it. Society and the media have done a great disservice to women by presenting them with only one version of the female image—the fashion model. There is no doubt that many of the professional models we see in the magazines and on television are attractive.

They are. I believe we should enjoy these photographs of models wearing beautiful clothes and exuding elegance, sexiness, and style. I also think, however, that women should learn to enjoy them with an *educated* eye, understanding and appreciating them for what they are—perfectly fit, perfectly styled, perfectly retouched, edited, colorized, deblemished, reproduced images of females.

Having worked in New York in the fashion industry, I wish each and every one of you could have the benefit of seeing what I saw. Seeing the "before and after" of a professional fashion magazine shoot. Seeing the hours and hours of hair and makeup, meticulously applied, retouched and reapplied by the world's foremost makeup and hair stylists. The hours of lighting setup done in the studios of the greatest photographers, to ensure that the models have the benefit of perfect light. And I wish you could bear witness to the thousands of dollars spent retouching the photos. If a model has a blemish that shows up in a picture, a photo retoucher is paid to take it out. If the model's hips look a little too full on any given day, the retoucher can shave off inches with a single stroke. If her breasts photograph too small, a retoucher can draw in cleavage. A single image you see in the pages of a fashion magazine may reflect more than $50,000 in retouching.

In other words, what you see on the pages of fashion magazines is not real. It is a beautiful, expensive, reproduction and re-creation of a photo. These photographs are exponentially different from the photos we take of ourselves and our family and friends. These images of women have been conceived, set up, shot, processed, and edited with techniques and processes completely unavailable to you or me.

Enjoy these pictures. But do not judge or compare yourself in any way, shape, or form to these images.

When they are done well, they are stunning, provocative, exciting, sexy, interesting, and downright beautiful. But learn to *balance* their importance in your life and the effect on how you view your own body. You now have the information you need to look at them with an educated, reality-based eye instead of with longing, jealousy, or idealization.

What the media show us is only a very narrow view of the actual body types that exist. By practicing your observation and awareness skills you will be delighted and enchanted by the beauty you find in a multitude of body types . . . a perfect balance of big, small, and everywhere in between.

2. BALANCE YOUR PRECONCEIVED IDEAS:
EVERYONE HAS AN ISSUE WITH THEIR WEIGHT.

It's just the way it is. Ask around. Thinking, talking, and obsessing about weight are a national pastime. It's the popular topic of the day. Women discuss it. Magazines debate it, surveys reveal it. Everyone, but everyone, has some weight-related issue. It transcends size. Thin women are just as obsessed (if not more) as well-rounded women. In fact, the more women I talk to about this book, the more I hear the same answer from our size 8 and size 10 sisters. The reaction is always the same when I ask if they are satisfied with their bodies. The answer is an identical "no" whether they are wearing a size 6 or 16 or 26.

Everyone has something that they want to change about their body. For years, I could never understand how a seemingly "thin" friend would moan and groan about struggling to lose those darn ten pounds. Hearing that made me want to *scream* because I was constantly at battle with my own darn *100* pounds. But through further discussion and in-depth questioning I came to discover something very important. Those ten pounds that my "thin" friends were battling could be just as emotionally debilitating to their lives as my 100 pounds were to mine. There is no difference in the self-esteem issues that live behind the weight. On that front, we are all equal. It doesn't matter if you are a size 2 or 22. We are all taught to feel inadequate about our bodies no matter what size or shape body we possess.

Society and the media beat all of us down, whether we know it or not, by showing us unrealistic images of women and then offering us close to 40 billion dollars' worth of diet and exercise options to "fix" ourselves. Additionally, the cosmetic surgery industry is steadily gaining popularity as another panacea for the imperfect body. The very sad fact of the matter is that the majority of women believe that their bodies are substandard in some way, shape, or form. Most women feel inadequate about their bodies because they think that they have something they need to fix.

The stories are endless. You know them as well as I do. Stories of women who will do anything to be on a diet, stick to a diet, lose weight, be thin. In our culture it is acceptable to starve ourselves, work out to levels of exhaustion, and even stick our fingers down our throats to get or stay thin.

Thinness. Everyone is obsessed with it. I run across women all the time who have tortured, fractured, weight-obsessed lives. And many of them are not what you or I would call "big." For instance:

I was away recently on a business trip staying in a full-service hotel. I decided after a long day to go to the health club and take a sauna to relax. There were several other women in with me. I was enjoying the peace and quiet when I noticed that one woman, very slight of frame, and with very little visible body fat, kept exiting the sauna every minute or two, rushing out for no more than thirty seconds, and then rushing back in again. In and out. In and out. In and out. Perhaps she got too hot and had to keep going out for air, I thought to myself. After ten or fifteen minutes, I left the sauna to jump in a cool shower, and as I did so, I paused and watched this woman quickly do one of her frequent exits from the sauna. She dashed out and headed straight for the scale. Jumping on, she read the number to herself, gave a pained look, and ran back into the sauna. I waited to try and digest what I had just witnessed and within a minute she was exiting the sauna again and replaying the whole weigh-in routine.

I realized that she was trying to see a decrease in the number on the scale by sweating in the sauna. Didn't she know that it was just water weight? Sweat? And the moment she drank a glass of water, it would go up again? She was a slave to a number on the scale, and would use any means to receive the "gratification" of seeing a magic number. I felt sorry for her. I wished I could have told her about the real-life gratification of learning to live gracefully in the body she has.

Or how about this one? Recently, at a luncheon, I sat next to an attractive woman in her late twenties. Although I don't remember her name, I'll call her Sarah. Sarah told me she worked for a political marketing group. She was tall and rather pretty, wearing what I guessed to be about a size 12. A very fit size 12. During the course of the lunch, the discussion turned to weight, dieting, etc. Sarah mentioned that she was envious of the body of a well-known actress whose photograph (modeling a string bikini) had recently appeared in *Vogue*. Now, you must know, the actress we were discussing is five feet two or three inches and weighs about 100 pounds wringing wet. She has a small frame, small bones, and is, generally, *small*. She was born that way. However, Sarah kept saying, "I am going to have a body just like hers and look like that in a bikini."

Well, I couldn't contain myself. I gently and lovingly tried to explain to Sarah exactly how *incredibly* impossible that would be, considering her body type was *radically* different from that of the actress in question. I further went on to explain that no matter how many step-aerobics classes she took, or how few calories she ingested, that she could never, *ever* achieve the same body as the actress. I closed my little monologue by saying how beautiful I thought Sarah's big, strong, healthy body was and that she should celebrate the body she has. Her reaction? She folded her napkin, pushed back from the table, slung her purse over her shoulder, and left.

I thought I was being helpful. But what I realized from this incident was how deep-seated weight issues run, not only in "big" women but within the Sarahs of the world as well. In spite of the fact that Sarah had a perfectly "acceptable" body, looked good in clothes, and was obviously an educated businesswoman, she had severe body-image insecurities that dominated her life.

Weight preoccupation is universal. Balance your belief that only we, as women of size, are weight conscious. It's just not true. Weight and body-image concerns and obsessions are common denominators among all women (and men too.) By recognizing that I was not alone, balancing in my own mind that millions of women of all shapes and sizes shared the same feelings, I didn't feel as alone and stranded in my own body. As a result, I could move forward and create for myself a healthy, happy, well-rounded outlook about my own body.

3. BALANCE YOUR REACTION TO NORMAL BODY FLUCTUATIONS: THEY ARE NATURAL AND SHOULD BE EXPECTED AS PART OF A HEALTHY, FUNCTIONING BODY.

Okay. Here's the deal. Our weight will *always* fluctuate. Day to day. Moment to moment. Research shows that normal daily fluctuations can range anywhere from one to six pounds on any given day, depending on the individual. This is true for everyone, whether we weight 120, 220, or 320 pounds.

For example, I recently returned from a friend's wedding. It was wonderful and I had a ball seeing old friends and enjoying all the festivities. Being away from home and my usual routine, naturally my eating habits changed as well. Instead of my usual "bread, veggies, fruit, chicken/fish and low-fat food" routine, I was having wedding cake, hors d'oeuvres, sauces, more wedding cake, champagne, diet Coke, crepes, and more wedding cake. After a wonderful weekend, and back home again on Monday, my body woke up feeling a little tired and bloated. My rings wouldn't fit on my fingers, and my face felt puffy. This is only natural, considering the foods I had been eating for the past two days.

Now there were two routes to take at this point. I could either feel guilty, wallow in it, stay inside, feel guilty, keeping eating, keep eating, keep eating, and let the temporary "condition" take over my otherwise normal Monday. That is what I would have done in the past. I decided to try a different tack. I decided to acknowledge that my body felt different than usual, *accept* the fact, and move on. I balanced the importance of the fluctuation—flowing *with* it instead of working against it. I got dressed, wearing something that I knew would feel comfortable and look good, put on my makeup, ate my usual fare, and got on with it. By the end of the next day, my body had readjusted and felt "normal" once again.

We all have times, occasions, holidays, evenings or weekends . . . vacations or honeymoons, or any number of other circumstances when our eating patterns are disrupted or altered. What is important, however, is learning to deal with our body's day-to-day natural fluctuations based on how we slept, how we feel, if we are getting sick, if we have PMS, if we had salty or spicy food, or any number of other normal daily occurrences. Our weight will fluctuate up and down a couple of ounces (or even pounds) on any given day. This is to be expected.

Successfully changing your life means knowing how to deal with your day-to-day fluctuations in weight, working *with*, not against them, and looking and feeling great no matter what.

In spite of any number of factors that can, and do, come into play on any given day, there have been times in my life when I *panicked* if I woke up feeling heavier than the day before. I imagined I was on an "upward spiral," pushing further and further up the scale, when, in fact, I was merely experiencing a slight, temporary body fluctuation. Out of fear and stress, I would eat my way toward oblivion, figuring why not? In my mind, if I woke up feeling "fat," I might as well go for it and eat more until I couldn't feel anything anymore, further alienating myself from hearing the natural rhythm of my body's ebbs and surges.

These days I practice a new routine. I practice an ongoing dialogue with my body. On any given day, these are the types of "balance" dialogues I have with my body:

- "I feel heavier today, and I acknowledge that feeling, allowing myself to experience it completely and calmly, knowing it is only temporary."
- "I understand that my body has natural weight fluctuations due to any number of normal physiological circumstances, and I will adjust and balance my day's activities accordingly, being mindful to take *extra* good care of myself, until I feel better."
- "Instead of beating myself up about the way my body feels today, I choose to pamper my body, slowly, lovingly, and approvingly flowing with the fluctuations, knowing they are temporary."
- "I will concentrate on conducting business as usual, accepting my natural fluctuation in weight."
- "I trust that my body is big, strong, healthy, and resilient, and will naturally readjust when it is ready to do so."
- "I accept that my body is a perfect machine. It shifts, grows, balances, adjusts, and readjusts naturally and effortlessly, adapting easily to my ever-changing daily needs and circumstances."

Balance is the acceptance that no two days are ever going to be the same. Our lives, like our bodies, are continually changing, growing, and evolving. Fluctuations in *all* areas of our lives (including our weight) are *normal*, and to be expected. *Balance* is the means by which we learn to live gracefully with those fluctuations.

Day-to-day fluctuations in weight are normal. Balance their importance in your life. Practice not overreacting or underreacting. Don't panic if your skirt is loose one day and tight the next. Instead, talk your body lovingly *through* the fluctuations—pamper and nurture instead of punish and condemn. You will be astounded how quickly you will feel your self again (and even better!).

Balance your life and your perception of your body using the three concepts given above. Don't expect every day to be picture perfect. Balance is the acceptance that no two days are ever going to be the same. Balance means that you are keeping your expectations in check and your preconceived notions at bay. And, most importantly, remember that there are going to be days when your skirt will be tight, when you eat more than your body needs, and when you feel downright cranky, sad, and blue. Learn to balance and accept these feelings, acknowledging them and allowing yourself to break down every once in a while.

I have bad days like everyone else, sad moments, when I'm feeling emotional and blue. Just ask my friend (and team member!) Malissa. She knows them all because she is usually the first person I call when insecurity creeps in every now and again. This is, in fact, a great time to call upon one of your team members. Malissa hears me out, listening to each and every word, and then somehow, miraculously, she makes me laugh. Use your team to help pull you through a bad day or a bad moment. You will feel better, and so will they for having been able to help you through a rough spot.

To *balance* ourselves is to expect the tumbles, the mishaps, and the gaffes, and learn to *mix them happily* with the rest, the good things that we experience. So often we have expected and anticipated a perfect time or weight somewhere far off in the future . . . a day when everything will be okay. For so long we have been told that we are not okay as we are and, as a result, we tend to live for the day when we are thinner. Balance teaches us to find the "okay" in *today*.

Balance the steps I am giving you. Don't try to gobble them all up at once. Some days will be better to try a relaxation session, some will be better for choosing new accessories for your uniform. One day you will feel like clearing the clutter from your closet, the next you will want to make time for moving your body. These steps are a "user's manual" for your well-rounded body, but don't forget that *you* are the user—with special needs and circumstances. Balance and mold the steps to fit your body and your life.

Believe

Negative feelings about our weight causes women to throw in the towel and stop believing in themselves. We are bombarded by the media with the single message "*be thin*." We are given a variety of ways to achieve this, each option more damaging to our self-esteem than the next.

These "options" we are given include compulsive dieting, fasting, taking pills, engaging in grueling and sometimes dangerous workouts, or even having surgery in order to change the way our bodies look. Is it any wonder that we have lost sight of the ability to truly believe in ourselves?

To *believe* is to validate one's own worth. I work every day to sustain a healthy sense of self-worth through daily *affirmations*. An affirmation is a statement made to oneself either aloud or silent, or sometimes written. An affirmation places a single, positive thought or idea into our conscious and subconscious minds and, with repetition, reinforces it. Affirmations support our beliefs. Affirmations are also very powerful. They have the ability to turn a "wish" into a reality. Remember the saying "Be careful what you wish for, because you might get it"? Affirmations are stronger than wishes. They are the creation of our reality in our mind.

I use positive affirmations all the time, but especially when my belief in myself starts to falter a little. It's the best pick-me-up I know. In fact, I keep a small notebook in my purse in which I write affirmations as I think of them. When I focus my mind on a single positive thought or goal, I remember and strengthen my belief in myself. For example, if I am having a difficult or stressful day, I might write an affirmation like this in my notebook ten or twenty times: "I feel relaxed, confident, and happy with myself in spite of any negative circumstances or situations I might come into contact with today."

Affirmations are tools that keep your beliefs alive and well and your self-worth in good shape. Here are some beliefs and affirmations to refer back to whenever you doubt the beauty of your own well-rounded body.

- *Believe in your new steps.* With a new set of guidelines to follow, your success will no longer be measured by how much you weigh. Losing weight is incidental to the process, merely the by-product of your positive feelings about your well-rounded body. Use the new steps when you feel like it and in your own way. *Affirmation:*

*These steps will serve as guidelines, helping me to live grace-
fully and joyfully inside my body. I will use the ones that are
right for me. I will tailor the steps to my own life and my own
body. The steps will teach me to celebrate all the wonderful
things I have to offer and share my confidence with my family,
friends, other well-rounded women, and the world.*

- *Believe that weight is not the source of all your problems.*
  Weight no longer has to be the overwhelming factor of
  your existence or hold you back from loving yourself
  any longer. In the ongoing process of changing, learning, and growing, real-life issues other than your
  weight will surface, and you will begin to deal with
  them one by one, and in your own time and way. As
  you make magnificent strides in how you think about
  your weight, you will find more and more "space" in
  which to work on other situations within your life. *Affirmation: I have started to realize that my worth is not based
  on my weight. I will take the time and space to think carefully
  about those areas of my life that need work. I deserve to be
  surrounded by beauty and joy, and choose to spend my time
  with supportive and loving people.*

- *Believe you have the power and strength to begin today.* So
  often we give up the power to change by making excuses. We relinquish the inner strength we all possess
  and fall into the old "I'm fat, I'm worthless" cycle, further delaying immediate positive change. You can
  change your whole life starting right now. Right this
  very second. And you do *not* have to lose weight to do
  it. All it takes is a decision in your own mind to accept
  instead of reject your own body. Once you do that, I
  will help you do the rest through the remaining steps.
  *Affirmation: Starting right this second, I choose to love myself
  as I am. I cannot and will not wait one more minute to begin
  loving my body as it is today. I can employ immediate changes*

in the way I feel about myself. I have decided to like myself from this point forward.

You have now completed the first step. You are ready to move forward onto Step 2, where you will learn the power of taking special "relax time" just for you!

1. In learning how to balance your perception of beauty, start to notice that healthy, beautiful bodies come in all shapes and sizes.

Be a body watcher. Practice looking at all sorts of bodies and noticing their individual qualities and attributes. Notice that no two are ever the same.

2. Take your own survey. Ask women of all shapes and sizes how they feel about their bodies. How many of them say they love their bodies just the way they are right now?

3. Notice and record how your body feels for five consecutive days. Does it feel exactly the same every day? How or how not? To what, if anything, can you attribute the fluctuations?

4. Bolster your belief in yourself by creating affirmations of your own. Keep a small notebook with you at all times and write affirmations when you need them.

If an individual is
able to love productively,
he loves himself too;
if he can love only others,
he cannot love at all.

—ERICH FROMM

STEP

2

Make Time

to

Relax

*R*elax. We hear the word all the time, but what does it really mean? How does it pertain to our busy lives? Relaxing means different things to different people, but the definition of relaxation that I want to explore here is *the conscious process of calming the mind and the body in order to reclaim the true self.*

Relaxation is not sleeping, watching television, or reading a book—although these activities can be preludes to relaxation. Relaxing is an independent activity in and of itself, something you schedule time to do during your day. Relaxation is an appointment you make to reclaim yourself. Relaxation works to relieve stress because it is virtually impossible to be relaxed and "stressed" at the same time.

"But who has time to relax?" you may be asking. We *all* have too many things to do and people, places, and situations that demand our attention. There are memos to write, meals to prepare, presentations to give, and children to be attended to. Our lives are increasingly more complex and complicated. The very real fact is that we are busy women with busy lives and with the pace of today's world, our responsibilities are rapidly expanding.

Being Everything to Everyone

Trying to "do it all" or "be it all" is a condition that I have found to be especially prevalent among women of

53

size. In fact, I was one of those who tried to do *everything* for *everyone else* except myself. I was the ultimate care-taker—fixing, mending, and solving the crises of others, all the while neglecting the one person who needed me the most. Me.

I began ignoring my own needs at an early age and first noticed it while in college. At the young age of nine-teen or twenty, instead of taking time and space to evalu-ate my own needs, I took on the role of "mom" to most of my college friends—doing and being all for everyone else. Need a ride? Catherine will take you. Struggling with a term paper? Ask Catherine to help you. Assistance tying the bow at the back of your formal party dress? Let Catherine do it. I took upon myself a number of tasks, roles, and duties in an effort to avoid taking the time and space to look at myself. I consciously put off my own needs (they were less important because I was fat) and took on responsibilities of others. It was one way to feel appreciated. But in the end, I was left alone, spent and sad. Everyone else was taking care of themselves—getting things done, going to parties, having an active extracur-ricular life—and I was left in dire need.

It is so easy to give ourselves away to others without taking care of our own needs first. Giving every last ounce of ourselves away is an excuse for not wanting to face our deeper issues of self-esteem and self-worth. *"I'm too busy to take care of me . . . I have to take care of [the kids, my mother, my husband, my boyfriend, the house, the people who work for me, etc.]* As women of size living in a "pro-thin" society, we have spent years being *ashamed* of our size, and as a result we try to compensate by putting the emphasis on *others* rather than on *ourselves*. We act for everyone else's benefit, hoping that it will "make up" or "cover up" for our shortcomings, namely, our weight.

54

It doesn't work. When you spend your life giving yourself away to others without taking the time to repair and renourish yourself you will find yourself in a state of emotional and physical exhaustion—feeling used, spent, and lonely. In fact, we cannot effectively and productively take care of those we love until we learn to take care of ourselves first. Taking time for ourselves in the form of relaxation is an integral step toward improved self-esteem.

Relax, Renourish, Reclaim

These are the three magic words. The moments we take for ourselves can lead to inner healing and self-acceptance. By scheduling and taking time for ourselves in the form of relaxation we are telling the world, "I am important and I deserve the time and space to renourish and reclaim my self." Unless we know how to keep ourselves intact, we are useless not only to ourselves but to others as well.

Remember back to a time when you were completely "stressed out." Think how you were being pulled in a thousand different directions, owing people time, money, or goods and services . . . trying to please everyone all at once and having to fix dinner at the same time!!! I would be willing to bet that at those moments (and we all have them) that you were not taking even as few as two or three minutes for yourself to relax, regroup, and reclaim. Just a few moments of *internal calmness* can clear your head, focus your attention, and rejuvenate your spirit.

Ask yourself this question right now. Am I taking the time necessary to work on myself from the *inside*? Do I allow myself the all-important moments of relaxation that I need to soothe and regenerate those parts of myself that I give so freely to others?

Relaxing allows time for the mind to quiet down if only for a few moments. When the mind is quieted, one is better able to hear all those important "signals" we talked about earlier—signals of what your body needs to eat, how it needs to move, and when it needs to rest. Profound thoughts and elusive crossword puzzle words alike will find their way into the *still* mind, where they might be cramped or pushed out of a crowded one.

Where and When to Relax

Relaxation happens *anytime* and *anywhere* you choose. That's the beauty of it. It requires no special equipment other than a quiet space. A few moments of complete relaxation is the best panacea for an overwhelming, hectic day.

I begin and end every day with some sort of relaxation. These sessions I loosely schedule into my mornings and evenings and usually last anywhere from five to fifteen minutes. After the alarm goes off but before I get up from bed in the morning (usually before I even open my eyes!) I take some time to clear my head, slowly waking from the previous night's rest, and preparing myself for a new day filled with new adventures and opportunities. I do the same in the evening before I go to sleep, quieting my mind, lovingly revisiting the day's events and preparing for a good night's rest.

At any given time during the course of my day, I might take one or a few unscheduled relaxation breaks, which I call daytime refreshers. Lasting usually one or two minutes each, these moments help me clear the clutter from my mind, regroup my thoughts, and repair any "damage" that might have been incurred through the long, busy day.

Brief periods of relaxation during the course of the day can also improve study time or pre-presentation jitters as they allow new information the *time* and *space* to assimilate into our consciousness. If you find yourself in a situation where you have already reached your "breaking point" or "boiling point," you have waited too long to relax. Try to get into a habit of taking a few moments to relax every day. Even if it's only one or two minutes, do it regularly and you will discover that you "break down" or "blow up" less and less frequently. The few moments you take to yourself are the easiest way to prevent "losing your cool."

Getting You Started with Your Breath

There is no right or wrong way to relax. If there were, it wouldn't be relaxation. How you choose to relax is entirely up to you! I will share some simple relaxation exercises that will get you started, but first let's take a moment to talk about breathing.

As you will come to see for yourself, focusing on your breath is one of the most effective ways to access a state of relaxation quickly. Our breath is the transportation that delivers us into a more relaxed state of being. Each breath that you take, and actually *notice* as you are taking it, will lead you into a deeper and more intensified level of relaxation.

Practice taking a few deep breaths right now. Inhale so deeply that you feel air travel through your nose and mouth down through your lungs and into your belly. Now, as you exhale, reverse the process and let your breath empty completely from your belly first, expelling next through the lungs and lastly through your nose or mouth. Do this several times, noticing the course your breath takes as it moves *down and in* and *up and out* of your body. Think about the inhale and the exhale equally.

Breathing is the cornerstone of effective relaxation. The more you are able to focus your awareness on your breath, the more relaxed you will become.

Three Relaxations for You to Try

Let's start with a morning relaxation. This is a good way to start your day. Maybe you will want to do a version of this relaxation every morning or perhaps just on the mornings when you have a "big day" in front of you. A morning relaxation can set the positive tone for the rest of your day!

Begin by finding a position wherever you are comfortable. Take several deep breaths, allowing your breath to slow down and even out. Notice both the inhale and the exhale equally as they move in and out of your body. As you are concentrating on your breath, allow any other thoughts you might be having to move aside gently, if only for the moment. Let all of the thoughts that surface—the invited ones as well as the "uninvited" ones— move through your consciousness with ease, neither encouraging nor stifling them. Concentrating back to your breathing will help clear your mind of other thoughts.

After you have become completely relaxed and are concen-

trating calmly on your even, slow breathing, begin to acknowl-edge the new day you are about to begin. Spend a moment recognizing how wonderful it is to be looking forward to a whole new day filled with new adventures and new opportunities. In your mind, walk through each of the coming day's activities, re-membering as closely as you can what they will be. Start with the activity you will be doing after you finish this relaxation. Take each of the planned activities and see it to fruition in your mind exactly as you desire it to unfold.

Envision yourself eating your breakfast and having it nour-ish you and give your body the energy it needs to begin the day. See yourself at the office, relating productively and pleasantly with your coworkers. Picture that very difficult meeting you might have to attend and see it unfold exactly as you would wish it to be. Go through as much of the coming day as you can, creating it in your relaxed and calm mind.

When you are finished "creating" your day, take a moment to bless every part of the coming day's events. Send a "blessing" ahead to each of your day's situations or locations. Send special blessings to those whom you will encounter during the course of the day who might try to cause you trouble or discomfort. Bless-ing these people and situations ahead of time protects and pre-pares you in advance from what the day might bring. It's preventive medicine of the best kind!

After you "create" your day in your relaxed mind, I want you to gently turn your focus to your own body and its miracu-lous daily functioning. Slowly go over in your mind each part of your body, relaxing it further. Begin at the top of your head and move slowly downward, taking a few moments to love, heal, and nourish each and every part. Take time to marvel at the beauty and ease with which your body operates so efficiently and so effec-tively for you.

As you complete your head-to-toe body awareness, repeat in your own mind any body-positive statement or group of state-

ments you choose, such as, "I love and approve of my body as it is this very day"; "I celebrate my beautiful body and all it does for me every day"; "I will spend today accepting my body just as it is, and loving every part of it for allowing me to move, breathe, love, and live"; "Today I will move and nourish my body in ways that make it feel wonderful." Spend time reflecting on these wonderful body-positive statements and letting them soak into your relaxed mind.

Slowly, and with a relaxed, positive mind, begin to bring your awareness back into the present day, time, and space. Feel the bed (or chair) beneath you and begin to hear the sounds of the morning—perhaps the birds outside, or others in your household awakening. Give yourself a few moments more to acclimate to the morning and then slowly open your eyes, feeling completely refreshed and ready to awake, arise, and begin your wonderful new day!

After your day is complete it's time to treat yourself to an evening relaxation. Taking the time to relax completely before you sleep allows you to quiet and clear your mind, preparing for a wonderful night of reparative rest.

Again, begin this relaxation by finding a position that is comfortable. Take several deep breaths, allowing your breath to slow down and even out. Notice both the inhale and the exhale equally as they move in and out of your body. As you are concentrating on your breath, allow any other thoughts you might be having to move aside gently, if only for the moment. Let all of the thoughts that surface—both the invited ones and the "uninvited" ones—move through your consciousness with ease, neither encouraging nor stifling them. Concentrating back to your breathing will help clear your mind of other thoughts.

After you have become completely relaxed and are concentrating on your even, slow breathing, begin to acknowledge the day you have just completed. As you calmly reflect upon the day's events, you might realize that you had, in fact, a terrific day. On the other hand, you might have had a very stressful one. Regardless of whether it was good, bad, or somewhere in between, the time has come to put it in its proper place—the past—and prepare for restful sleep before you begin a new day.

Spend a few moments giving closure to each of the day's events. Go through them briefly in your mind and, without re-opening or actively revisiting any of the events in a stressful way, gently cover them with a "blanket of acceptance." Don't try to force, change or alter what occurred, just bless it, close it, and move on.

After you have put healing and closure on the past day, you can ready your body for sleep. Slowly go over in your mind each part of your body, relaxing it further. Begin at the top of your head and move slowly downward, taking a few moments to love, heal, and nourish each and every part. Take time to reflect on the beauty and ease with which your body operated so efficiently and so effectively for you all day long. As you visit and further relax each body part, thank it for all the work it has done for you. For example, thank your eyes for guiding you through your day with clarity of vision; your lungs for pumping glorious air in and out of your body, keeping you alive by your breath; your arms for their strength and agility of movement, allowing you to carry boxes, drive a car, wave at your neighbor, hug your children, and so on.

Take a few extra moments to linger on body parts that may be ailing or perhaps just a little under the weather. If you had a sore neck all day, take time to make sure it is completely relaxed and resting in a natural, comfortable position. Send positive energy and thoughts to that area of your neck, asking it to heal itself overnight. I sometimes use the power of color in healing relaxations all over my body. I do this by sending a "shot" of a single color to areas of my body that need some extra attention.

The color you choose is entirely up to you. Just think about it for a brief moment, and a color will pop into your mind. That is the color to use at that time. Send a "bolt" (or a "cloud") of the most vibrant intensity of that color to the specific body area. Envision the color moving in and around the body part, washing away pain, stress, or illness, replacing it with the clean, clear intensity of that color.

As you complete your head-to-toe body relaxation, repeat in your mind a final body-positive statement or group of statements that you choose to fall asleep with, such as, "I will go to sleep tonight and awake tomorrow accepting my body just as it is, and loving every part of it for allowing me to move, breathe, love, and live."

A Daytime Refresher is any relaxation done during the course of the day, at the spur of the moment, on a *need-to-do* basis. Daytime refreshers are moments of unscheduled relaxation that you take when things are getting hurried, hectic, or chaotic. A few, very brief moments of relaxation for yourself will calm your mind, clear your head, and collect your thoughts. Close your office door, take the phone off the hook, or ask your neighbor to watch your kids for five minutes.

Close your eyes while taking several deep breaths. Make sure each breath reaches all the way down to your lower belly on the inhale, and pushes completely out of your nose or mouth on the exhale, leaving the belly empty of air. Pick a word, any word, and begin to say it over and over in your head, coordinating your breathing with the sound of the word. I sometimes choose the word "relax" or "focus" and repeat it in my head taking the inhale to say "re-" (or "fo-") and the exhale to say "-lax" (or "-cus"). You can choose any word you wish, but pick what I call a "benign" word, one that won't cause anxiety or stress when you say it to yourself.

After you have gotten more deeply relaxed by your breathing and thinking of your word, picture that relaxed feeling you have right now permeating everything you are doing, touching, seeing, or hearing. Let the soothing vibrations coming from this calm, rhythmic sensation expand outward around your desk, your office, your home, or wherever you might be at the moment.

Let the peaceful vibration radiate outward from your body, washing over everyone you will come into contact with for the rest of the day. See the calm, centered feeling moving into spaces and places you will have to be before the day is out—in your car, in the grocery store, or in a meeting. See the calm, easy, relaxed feeling have a life of its own—radiating outward from your body and into your world.

Take a few more deep breaths while again repeating your word of choice, and slowly begin to focus your awareness back to your immediate surroundings. Begin to hear the noises and the sounds around you. Feel the weight of your body in the chair where you are seated. Slowly open your eyes and prepare to reenter the day with a newfound inner calmness and clarity of mind.

These are only three basic examples of relaxation exercises you might choose to do. Feel free to expand on them, incorporating the most effective imagery for you. These are merely guidelines to get you in to the habit of making time for yourself in the form of gentle, reparative, rejuvenating relaxation. Once you get used to making the time and space to relax, you can use the relaxation periods to accomplish gentle and meaningful bodywork imagery as well. The one that follows is a great one to get you started!

Bodies in Space

This is a very good relaxation exercise for getting in touch with how your body fits into the landscape of the world. Women of size are often guilty of overestimating how much, or how little, space they occupy. I ask many of the women I work with to describe to me how they imagine their bodies fitting into the landscape of their world. Most women say things like, "I'm bigger than all my friends," or "My body is larger than my friend Jane's, but I'm still smaller than Rosemary," or "I wear a much bigger size than most of my friends," or "I weigh ten pounds more than I did five years ago," or "I'm much bigger since my second child was born," or even, simply, "I am *huge*." Although these comparisons are how we might *feel* about our bodies, they are actually very limited in their scope.

Most women tend to view their bodies in direct comparison to (a) other women's bodies; (b) how their bodies "used to be" at some other point in time; or (c) some other gross miscalculation dreamed up in their heads. These reference points are very limiting, as they tell us nothing about how our physical self relates to the world around us. I have found that it is very helpful to take a moment to step back and *view ourselves from a distance*, with a short but effective visualization. I want you to try to move away from your "self" and to imagine your body from several new vantage points.

First, sit in a comfortable chair and take a few deep breaths. Close your eyes and allow the darkness you "see" to become a luscious, velvety backdrop for this visualization exercise. In your mind's eye, I want you to look at yourself from afar. In other words, pretend you are someone else watching you. I want you to watch yourself as if you were watching someone in a movie.

See yourself as you are right now . . . look at yourself sitting in the room. Now take note of the scale of your body compared to the scale of the chair. What percentage of the chair do you occupy? Probably somewhere between 75 to 95 percent, depending on the size of the chair. Now back up farther and look at yourself in comparison to the size of the room. What percentage of the room do you occupy? If it's a very small room, maybe you take up 15 percent of it; otherwise maybe only 1 or 2 percent, or even less. Now picture your body as it relates to the size of the whole house or apartment building. See from a distance how small a percentage your body occupies—far less than 1 percent, right?

Now back up even farther. In your mind, "fly" up in the sky and see how your body looks in relation to the size of the town in which you live. (Remember, you are still looking at yourself sitting in that chair.) As you look at the bird's-eye view of your city, your body as it sits in that chair will look amazingly small . . . just a tiny dot on the map. Take your "flying" up even farther and try to see your body sitting in the chair as you look at the earth from space. It is impossible. The size of your body is completely inconsequential compared to the space around you in the universe.

Now "fly" back down into your country, your state, your city, and your house. Bring yourself back to the room where you are sitting and back into your "self." Slowly become aware of being back inside your body, feel your feet on the floor, and notice where your hands are resting. Open your eyes and breathe.

The purpose of this visualization exercise is to expand your points of reference for your body. Sizewise, your body can be compared to any number of things, and what you will discover is that it is *smaller* than most of the points of comparison you come up with. It is sometimes helpful for women to reassess how they view their body, recognizing that it is larger than some things in the world, and smaller than others. The trick is to see our body from as many different vantage points as possible—with no particular one being "right" or "wrong." Our body is just one of the infinitesimal elements in space.

As you have now seen, you can easily adapt your relaxation sessions to explore issues about your own body.

Three Big Tips for Living a More Relaxed Life

1. Slow down. We live in a society where everyone is in a hurry. When you are in a stressful situation or caught up in the heat of the moment, *slow down* and *ease up* a little. What you will find is that the process of slowing down will allow you the time and space to think more clearly, without being additionally pressured by the rush, rush, rushing. When you are thinking more clearly you can better focus on the situation at hand and attend more carefully to all the details. Slowing down will also help you prioritize what's really important and what can wait.

One sure way to get yourself to slow down a little is to take short relaxation breaks whenever you feel pressured or stressed. A moment or two of quiet relaxation will quiet your mind and automatically slow you down, clear your head, and refocus your attention.

2. Live in the present. We all have the tendency to live for some "magic moment" in the future. As a woman of size, I spent many years anticipating the day when I

would be thin, and I pinned all my hopes and dreams and aspirations on that day. I denied the beauty of the present moment and lived in expectancy of the day my life would come together because I would be thin. Ridiculous. Think of how much valuable and precious time that wastes.

Living in the present means living in the here and now—this day, this hour, this moment. It involves a conscious decision to pay more attention to each experience rather than looking forward to "better" experiences in the future. You will find it easier to be relaxed when you start to live in the moment instead of living for the future. When you really think about it, all we have in life is an extensive collection of individual moments. Why not try to enjoy each and every one of them instead of putting life off until a "better" moment arrives? True relaxation and long-lasting inner calm are achieved by acknowledging and celebrating the here and now.

3. Surround yourself with positive people. Take a moment to inventory the people in your life. What type of people are they? Happy? Fulfilled? Do they see the glass as half empty or half full? Learning to take time for yourself and to take care of yourself is easier when you surround yourself with people who do the same. Work on cultivating friendships and acquaintanceships with those who are loving and accepting not only of you but of themselves as well. Banish negative, bitter, unhappy people from your life. Devote time to those who lift you up, not bring you down.

Learning to take time for yourself is crucial in the process of becoming well rounded. Once we know how to allow ourselves time and space for our own thoughts and needs, we can effectively begin changing our lives for the better.

Now that you have started to reclaim some time for yourself, let's move on and begin an exciting new relationship with your own body!

1. Do you take the time to relax, renourish, and reclaim yourself? If so, describe when, where, and how. If not, list below the potential times and places during your day where you could find room for relaxation.

_____

_____

_____

2. Which parts of your day do you find that you most want a few relaxing moments to yourself?

_____

_____

3. Give one (or all) of the sample relaxations a try in your own time and your own way. Try at least one of them a day for several weeks and record changes you feel in the way you handle your life, your work, your family, your responsibilities.

4. Practice "present moment awareness"—living and experiencing each day, each moment, as it happens. Notice and record any changes you might notice.

5. List all the people in your life who lift you up. Make a commitment to see them or make contact with them more often.

The Human body, at peace with itself,
Is more precious than the rarest gem,
Cherish your body, it is yours this one time
  only.

The human form is won with difficulty.
It is easy to lose.
All worldly things are brief, like lightning in
  the sky.

Life you must know as the tiny splash of a
  raindrop:
A thing of beauty that disappears even as it
  comes into being.
Therefore, set your goal.
Make use of every day and night to achieve
  it.

—JE TSONG KAPA

Initiate a Relationship with Your Body

$\mathcal{S}$tep 3 is about reconnecting, rejoining, and revisiting an old relationship. Not with your sixth-grade crush, your long-lost cousin, or your college sweetheart, but with your very own body.

We all know what a relationship is, and we know what factors constitute a good one. For a good relationship we need trust, understanding, respect, clear communication, and love. All of these factors hold true for creating a relationship with our bodies as well.

What do I mean by a "relationship with our body"? I mean that we will be exploring the state of disrepair that exists between our heads and our bodies. After we examine where the relationship has gone astray, I will give you the tools and information you need to forge ahead and create a new, loving relationship with the body you have today.

Relationship: The Breakup

Women have learned to "break up" with their bodies for reasons of self-preservation. We are smart creatures and have discovered that in order to survive in a world filled with messages telling us that we will not be "real" people until we are thin, we have learned to dissociate our bodies from the rest of who we are. We become women living from our necks up. Yes, we are still mothers, wives, girlfriends, daughters, students, and executives, but we hold those titles *in spite of* our size, rather than *in celebration of* it.

73

Growing up large, I got the message through friends, family, teachers, and the media that by being big, I was being "bad." I was "misbehaving," not "minding," not being a "good girl." I was taunted, teased, and ridiculed for my generous body, being pushed further and further away from "connecting" with and learning how to accept and love it. Instead, I learned to associate my weight with my self-worth, and I found it increasingly difficult to learn to love and accept myself. My body was my battle-field *and* my enemy. Naturally, I sought ways to dissoci-ate myself from the one thing that was causing me the most pain—my body. So, at some point, although I can-not remember exactly when, I "broke up" with my body. Year by year I shut down more and more contact with my physical self. My size had become the primary source of shame, pain, anger, and guilt. I was still me . . . Catherine . . . but only Catherine from the neck up. A pretty face, shiny long hair, smart and funny. But anything below the neck I didn't address or acknowledge. I didn't look at my body, wouldn't touch it, wouldn't listen to it, wouldn't pamper or adorn it. I chose to ignore it altogether. The relationship with my body was over. Done. Finished.

My breakup began sometime during my adoles-cence, because I was a fat kid. But it can happen at any time. In the name of survival, to spare our dignity and self-worth, it becomes necessary to separate ourselves from the source of our pain, namely, our body. We begin to treat our body as an annoying appendage, a mass (or mess) of shame, and a constant reminder of how we have "failed." Our bodies become separate entities of foreign matter, completely unrelated to our lives.

Many women will recognize this phenomenon, the separation of the body from the *self*. It is a protection device we use to prevent from collapsing under the pressure we put ourselves through to fit society's image of how we *should* look. We learn to see ourselves only from the neck up, abandoning and alienating our bodies below the chin. Viewing ourselves only from this very limiting vantage is one of the key factors of the breakup with the rest of our bodies. Although done for reasons of self-preservation, breaking up with our body can be the most damaging breakup of our lives.

Relationship: The Makeup

The best part of breaking up is making up, right? In this step, you will begin to acknowledge the breakup and initiate the makeup with your body. Making up is not a one-time thing. We will begin to rebuild the foundation upon which your new relationship will rest. Our goal is to reestablish the connection with the body . . . the whole body, including torso, tummy, thighs, and hips. Everything. Your new relationship will be one based in trust, understanding, communication, and forgiveness. I will give you the information and guidance you need to approach your own body with love and understanding—forging the way for a new, healthy, hands-on relationship.

Crisis at Body Central

Women today are in a state of crisis with our bodies. We are at war with them. We constantly berate, compare, contort, and unnecessarily exhaust them—overcontrolling and forcing them into unnatural shapes, forms, and sizes. We beat, flex, and starve them. I have concerns for *all* women, not just women of size. The war with the

75

female body, trying to achieve unreal ideals shown in fashion magazines, is killing the natural female form. I like to describe the female body as "curvy," "strong," "rounded," "healthy," and "shapely." Don't those words sound more empowering and positive than "thin," "small," "reduced," and "slim"?

I recently received a letter from a friend of mine (a beautiful red-headed size 18) who is living abroad. She writes: "Did you know that in Morocco large-size women are called 'forte,' meaning 'strong'? Isn't that wonderful? A woman is beautiful because of her face. A large, healthy woman's body represents happiness. A voluptuous woman represents comfort, well-being, and joy to her family." She's right. "Forte" is a wonderful way to describe our bodies. They are big and strong. Strong enough to work and play and have babies. Strong enough to rearrange the living room furniture, carry groceries, and run after children. Strong enough to create an impact when we walk into a room. Strong enough to radiate beautiful, smart, vibrant energy in the workplace. Strong, big, powerful. Not weak, small, and frail.

Getting Comfortable

In order to live fully each and every day, we need to feel comfortable in the body we have. That means the body we have *right this minute*—not next week, next month, or five years ago. I don't intend for this to sound easy by any means. Very few women of any shape or size are able to say that they are happy inside their bodies. What a pity. There are so many wonderful aspects of our feminine shapes, and the breadth and width of diversity they encompass. There is so much to enjoy, and so much to celebrate.

Feeling comfortable means accepting—accepting and loving, inclusive of faults. This is a very difficult thing to learn to do. It's hard for all women, not just women of size. Give it a test. Ask anyone. Any woman. Any friend. Your neighbor. The lady checking you out at the grocery store. Your sister. Your son's teacher. See what they say when you ask if they are comfortable with their bodies. I can almost guarantee that the response the majority of women give will range from mild to severe *dissatisfaction*. You will hear things like, "I'm too fat." "I weigh too much." "My thighs are too big." "I hate my hips." "My stomach isn't flat." "My arms jiggle." "I have a flabby bottom." And on and on and on. Keep asking. You'll get a few "I'm too thin"s, but the majority of women you ask will say that they need to lose weight. My question for all these women is, by whose standards do they consider themselves "overweight"? Over *what* weight? The life insurance charts? Over *whose* weight? Supermodels? Neighbors? Relatives? The size they wore when they were twenty-one?

Getting comfortable inside the body you have today means you are able to say aloud to yourself, "I love and accept my body the way it is. Every part of it . . . every inch and every pound. I am making the conscious decision to quit punishing myself for my weight, and to start a loving, healthy relationship with the body I have." When you say these words (and you will!), you have reached a point that very few women of *any* size have reached.

You Must Remember This . . .

We are now into the actual work of rebuilding the relationship with our body. And to begin, I would like to share with you a single concept that has helped me to reapproach my body in a new manner. Acceptance of this is crucial to the healing of your relationship with your own body.

All positive change comes from self-love, not self-hatred. In order to initiate any sort of long-lasting and wonderfully positive change in our lives, we must do it because of *how much we like ourselves.* For instance: I believe that it is counterproductive to stand in front of a mirror and tell ourselves how much we hate our body. Negative complaining or obsessing about any situation—be it about our job, a relationship, or our body—will not lead to a positive solution.

We must practice loving respect of ourselves in order to turn a situation onto a positive course. Only when we realize and recognize our own uniqueness and self-worth can there be room for positive change to occur. Let me give you an example from my own experience.

My body settled in at its present size over a period of five or six years. And those five years directly coincide with the years I spent working in publicity for a wonderful children's television network. While working there, I experienced great boosts of self-esteem and positive surges of self-worth. Because of the work I was doing, and my love and respect for the people I was working with, I began to feel empowered and appreciated. I was part of a young, vibrant, creative team and felt wonderful about the work I was accomplishing.

It was during my four years there that I realized I was losing weight. *Without* dieting or obsessing, and over the course of four years, I inched down the scale from 265 to 215 pounds. As I look back, I attribute my drop in weight to the happiness and satisfaction I was feeling. Work was great and I was stimulated, confident, and relaxed with the life I had created for myself in New York. During that period, *my weight lost me* instead of the other way around. I genuinely liked and accepted myself, pleased with what I was doing and, as a result, my body adjusted itself accordingly.

Constantly find new ways to build yourself up— keep yourself feeling appreciated, trusted, and needed— whether that be through a work situation or personal relationships. Be your own best cheerleader. Seek out circumstances where you are valued and appreciated. Don't allow yourself to get stuck in situations that make you feel crummy about yourself. Banish negativity at all costs. Build an environment of self-love and self-approval. Surround yourself with loving, supportive people who accept you as you are today.

Change is a wonderful thing. It can help us to grow, learn, and evolve. Attempts to make positive changes from negative, self-hating, spiteful, jealous feelings are attempts made in vain. We are only able to make positive, loving, complete lasting change by loving and appreciating ourselves as we are.

Caution: Learning to like yourself is very powerful. The long-term feeling you experience by truly loving and accepting yourself is magical. You can move mountains. Loving yourself is an incantation and a spell that will work its magic in every area of your life. It's like having your own personal genie in a bottle. And the wonderful surprise is that the "genie" has been you all along!

Inner Assessment

Changing your life means being able to see yourself as a whole and complete human being. Most of who you *really* are has nothing to do with your weight. You are infinitely more than just your physical body. Who you are begins and ends on the inside. A great deal of time and energy should be spent on acknowledging, nurturing, and celebrating your *inner* assets—those things that you like about yourself—personality traits, good qualities, natural talents and abilities. Assessing your positives begins from the *inside*. Inner assets are those things that make you uniquely *you*!

Inner assessment can be easily broken down into two categories: Things you like about yourself ("I like X") and things you can do ("I can X"). These are two very powerful sentences—powerful words about yourself that have the potential to change your life.

The "I like" sentence urges you to remember all those things that you like about yourself. It can be as simple as *I like the way I relate so well to my kids. I like the fact that I can speak well in public. I like my strength. I like my sense of humor. I like being able to make people feel good about themselves. I like waking up happy every morning. I like my clarity and conciseness. I like my laugh. I like the way I sound when I sing in the shower.*

The "I can" statement is a powerful reminder of the multitudes of things you are able to do, and do well. For instance; *I can walk four miles. I can change a fuse in my car. I can move furniture around my house. I can write. I can hit a fantastic backhand in tennis. I can tell a good story or joke. I can make lunch for four screaming, hungry children in three minutes flat. I can play the piano.*

Assessment of our inner qualities and natural abilities acts as a reminder of all the things we do like about ourselves and all the things we *can* do. There is nothing more uplifting during a bad day or a frenzied moment than to take a break and build yourself back up from the inside.

I keep a beautiful crystal bowl in my office filled with little pieces of paper—each with one of my inner assets written on it. Whenever I am feeling blue, depressed, negative, or just a little blah, I reach in and pull out one of my inner assets and read it aloud (on a really bad day, I pull out two or three!). These are little reminders to keep myself focused on my positives and strengths—to stimulate a cycle of positive growth instead of becoming bogged down in negative thought patterns.

The Physical Relationship with Your Body

I have now shared with you the concepts that will help you create a new relationship with your body. Understanding and accepting these ideas will stimulate the process of reshaping your preconceived thoughts about your body and your weight.

It is now time to begin the "physical" part of the relationship with your body—practicing loving, hands-on rituals that increase body awareness and enhance overall well-being. Learning to love the touch and feel of the body you have is crucial in creating and maintaining a healthy, nurturing relationship with your body. These hands-on techniques I suggest will span your entire body, from hair to toenails, lavishing *attention* and *touch* to long-overlooked body parts.

Over time and due to the "neck up" syndrome explained earlier, women have neglected having physical contact with their bodies. For many years, I was scared to touch my body or lavish attention on any one part of it. In the shower, I would let the water do all the work, rarely or never allowing myself to really touch my own body. I would dress quickly, always mindful to cover myself completely and avoiding mirrors at all costs. Makeup, facials, manicures, massage, pedicures, and waxing were alien concepts—luxurious rituals reserved for the day when I was thin. Have I ever come a long way! Just last year, I was vacationing in Morocco where I enjoyed a beauty treatment at a *hamman*, a traditional Moroccan bathing establishment. After you pay a fee and strip down, you are scrubbed, loofahed, and invigoratingly washed head to toe by a hamman attendant who is trained to rub, clean, and polish you until you shine! This is a delight that I can barely describe in words, but one that for many years I would have avoided like the plague.

It took years, but slowly, and mostly through my work in the modeling world, I took a more hands-on approach with my body. I watched other models, listened to them talk, and watched how they did their hair and their makeup. I studied how they plucked their eyebrows and how they kept up with manicures and heard stories of massage therapy sessions.

Models of all shapes and sizes who rely on their bodies for their livelihoods are wonderful examples because they treat their bodies as precious objects—pampering, buffing, adoring, polishing, and perfecting every last inch. They know how to take care of their bodies, and by watching and listening and learning, I began my own regimen of hands-on care and upkeep for my body. Little by little I realized that the more positive body maintenance and grooming experiences I had, the more in tune I became with my own body, and the less I feared it. I began a lifelong physical relationship with my own body.

Eight Simple Steps
Hands-On Rituals

The remainder of Step 3 will consist of a few hands-on body ritual suggestions, ways I have discovered to pamper and celebrate the body today. The rituals will be broken down into the main areas of immediate disrepair—skin, feet and hands—and "challenging areas." Included in each are loving acts of care and grooming that will leave you feeling and looking your best. Try one. Try a few. Spend fifteen minutes a day trying new body-awareness rituals. In the process, you will probably come up with some rituals of your own.

SKIN

Skin includes every inch of flesh on our body. And we, as large-size women, have an abundance of "inches" to care for! If properly maintained, our skin should radiate good health and be soft to the touch. It's a gift—let's maximize it!

My skin-care mantra is simple: "hydrate, exfoliate, moisturize." Hydration of the skin comes from within—and this is achieved by drinking water as often as possible. Water keeps your skin soft and supple and helps to reduce drying, which can lead to wrinkling. Drink lots of water as often as you like. It doesn't matter what kind of water: bottled, distilled, sparkling, with or without "gas," as they say in Europe, or just plain old tap water. Out of fancy blue bottles, or leaning over the hose in the backyard, just drink it. Lots of it.

There are many theories on the correct amount of water one should drink, how it aids weight loss, burns fat, curbs appetite, etc., but I ignore all of that. Instead, I

83

seduce myself into finishing at least one 50-ounce bottle of water a day because of my skin. When I drink water, my skin looks better. I don't "break out" as often in the hot summer months, and in the winter my lips don't get dry and chapped.

Drinking water benefits your skin in three ways. First, it helps to flush out toxins that naturally build up inside your body and can lead to skin flare-ups and breakouts. Secondly, water actually "plumps" the skin's cells, hydrating them and creating a healthier, glowing complexion. And finally, drinking water prevents the skin from dryness—nourishing and hydrating the cells and stimulating the natural skin rejuvenation process.

Water reminds me of models and a secret I learned from them: models of all sizes—whether walking to and from jobs in NYC; backstage at the fashion shows in Paris and Milan; having fittings in designer's studios; having makeup applied before a photo shoot, or at an early morning runway show rehearsal—all models have a bottle of water within arm's reach wherever they go. If you were to ask them why, I can guarantee that they would answer, "For my skin." Call it a trade secret. But now you're in on it. Don't drink water to lose weight. Drink water to make your skin look beautiful. Hydrate from within.

Exfoliation comes next in my skin mantra. To exfoliate is to clean by removing the layers of dead skin. I like to gently help my skin "shed" as all skin naturally does, leaving behind a softer new skin surface. The trick to remember with exfoliation is that a little can go a long way. I remember days as a teenager, scrubbing my face raw with a "buff puff,' thinking that the harder I scrubbed, the better my skin would get. Wrong. Overscrubbing (overexfoliating) can lead to serious, sometimes permanent skin damage, especially on sensitive skin areas such as the face.

Of all areas of my body, I am most careful with the cleaning and exfoliating of my face. The skin on the face can be extremely sensitive, especially around the eye area, where the skin is "thinner." In addition to my daily cleansing routine, I find it beneficial to have a professional deep-cleaning, exfoliating, and hydrating facial once a month. If once a month is out of the question (as it sometimes is for me), then treat yourself to a professional facial whenever you are able. Twice a year is better than not at all. Your skin and face are worth the monthly investment (anywhere from thirty to sixty dollars) and the cumulative results will last a lifetime.

Before you begin your facial with a beauty esthetician, ask her what type of products she uses. You should know your own skin well enough to know what type of products will irritate it and what will not. I know that I have extremely fair, sensitive skin and that my face reacts violently to perfumed products. I ask, "Do any of the products you are going to use have perfume in them?" before every facial just to be careful.

If you are having a facial and something doesn't feel right—if it stings or feels overly irritating—don't be afraid to speak up. It's *your* skin, after all, and you are paying to keep it beautiful, not to irritate it. At some point during your professional facial, your esthetician will apply a "mask," or sometimes two, to your face. Depending on which type she uses (ask her—there are hundreds of different types) the mask will act as a skin exfoliator, skin normalizer, or skin rejuvenator.

Exfoliating doesn't stop at the face. For exfoliation of the rest of the body, I suggest setting up an exfoliation sanctuary near your bath or shower area. I have a basket

I keep at the side of my bathtub filled with sponges and loofahs of all shapes and sizes. While taking a few minutes to relax in the tub or sing in the shower, I grab one of my loofahs and gently scrub and rub all over my body, removing dead skin and deep-cleaning away the daily dirt. I suggest buying a loofah "mitt" that you wear on one of your hands, making it easy to control and maneuver over the sensuous curves and valleys of your body. Do not overscrub. Remember that your skin is tender and should be exfoliated with gentle, loving care, not overzealous aggression.

Moisturizing your skin is the final step in my skincare mantra. Moisturizing is actually hydration from the *outside*. When I was younger, I often shunned moisturizers, claiming that I had "oily" skin and didn't need them. I feared that creams and lotions would make me break out. What I have learned over the years is that *all* skin types need moisture and that there exists a wide variety of moisturizers available to suit any skin type. A good moisturizer can act as a protective layer from the elements such as dirt, grime, and most of all, the sun. Your skin's worst enemy is the sun. Believe me, this is difficult for me to write. I grew up in a sun-worshipping family in the days before skin cancer warnings. "Tan fat is better than white fat" was a favorite Lippincott household saying. Or "Let's go to the pool to *sunburn* for a while." Yikes. Aside from the very real and dangerous risk of sun-induced skin cancer, the sun beats up on your skin, causing unnatural dryness and premature wrinkling. How do you avoid seasonal derma disasters both winter and summer? By keeping your skin moisturized year-round, wearing a moisturizer that contains an active sunscreen (at least on your face) every day.

Obviously, there are many moisturizers to choose from and you may have to test a few before you find the one (ones) that are right for you and your skin type. I use different creams and moisturizers on different areas of my body and change them with the seasons. I use "lighter" lotions for summer (eucalyptus scent is one of my favorite summer cooling creams), and heavier-duty ones for harsh winter months. I have one for my face for day and one for overnight. And then I use another for my body after showering or bathing.

In the winter, I usually suffer chapped hands, so I have an intensive, thick cream just for that purpose. And I am the most religious (as you should be) about the tender eye area, keeping it well moisturized and reducing dryness and wrinkling. Every night before bed, I apply a moisturizing eye cream on the sensitive area around my eyes.

Your skin is the part of your body that is exposed most to the elements. Notice how much softer the "covered" areas of skin on your body are. Feel how soft your stomach or buttocks or underneath your upper arm are. Our exposed skin is abused daily from the sun, cold weather, pollution, and soaking up the dirt of daily life. Moisturizing helps to keep our overexposed areas looking their best.

HANDS AND FEET

The state in which we keep our hands and feet is in direct relation to how we feel about ourselves. If they are clean and well groomed, it is an indication that we feel confident about our appearance. If they are not, it is the first sign of a negative body image.

No matter what your size, your age, your shape, or your skin color, you can *always* have great looking, well-groomed hands and feet. It's a telltale sign that you care *about yourself.* Caring for your hands and feet doesn't mean that you have to have long, perfectly polished "superglam" nails. Caring means that you know your own lifestyle and what suits you best and you don't stretch your limitations.

Example: I have a friend who is a painter and refinisher of decorative furniture. She works with her hands all day long, exposing them to paints, varnishes, stains and heavy-duty paint removers. She knows that she cannot have long, high-maintenance nails. Instead, she keeps her nails short and natural colored. She uses moisturizers generously to combat the effects of all the paint products she works with daily.

On the other hand, my grandmother Mimi had beautiful long nails that perfectly set off her elegant hands. Based on her lifestyle (phone, poodles, and lunches) she wore fire-and-ice reds in the winter and coral pinks in the summer. Always perfect, long, and unchipped, she had the time to pamper and paint her nails regularly. I, however, do not.

For many reasons, I keep my nails short, with one coat of clear polish. In my heart of hearts, I would like to be a little more adventurous, but I choose to keep it simple based on my lifestyle as a model. And as a model, it is my job to make my body a blank canvas upon which a client (a store, a designer) can adorn me with their clothes and accessories in line with *their* vision, not mine. Painted nails detract from a blank canvas, and I don't have the time (or the patience) to constantly change my nail color. Result: I keep my nails short, clean, and clear. I have found this to be the easiest to maintain and work into my lifestyle. I do my nails myself and have a professional manicure about once a month. Here are some nail "tips" that work well for most beautiful but busy women of size.

- *Choose a polish color that is appropriate.* Bright reds or pinks might be fine for a dressy night out or on your toes during the summer, but may be less suited for the office. Stick to what is appropriate.

- *Keep your cuticles in shape.* Bitten, bloody, and ragged is not attractive.

- *Keep your nails "even" in length.* If one or several break, file them *all* down.

- *Use a "whitening pencil."* These inexpensive "pencils" are made to draw under the nail (like you are cleaning it) and leaves behind an extra "zing" of whiteness for enhancing natural nails.

- *Keep your nail polish chip free.* If it chips and you do not have time to fix it, take off *all* the polish.

Aside from your nails, your hands appreciate extra attention as well. Every so often, and usually during the winter months, I will give myself an overnight hand-conditioning treatment. I generously apply a heavy cream to my hands and don white cotton gloves. I sleep in the gloves, letting the cream soak into my dry hands. This treatment provides overnight relief from dry, rough hands.

These days, I notice that more and more women will spend a great deal of time and money on their nails. They have weekly manicures, nail bonding, nail tips, silk wraps, and nail extensions, spending hours of upkeep on their hands each month. And then I look at their feet. Disastrous! I say, spend half as much time (and money) on your nails and devote the rest to your feet!

Nothing is worse than seeing an otherwise luscious large-sized woman with uncared-for feet. The simple fact is that our feet end up taking the most abuse for carrying around our bigger, better bodies all day. We are more prone to calluses from our weight, and rashes from friction, heat, and sweat. Even if I have to dig change out of the car seat, I have a professional pedicure twice a month. For me, it is a necessity. I walk a great deal and my feet take the toll from it. Regular pedicures keep my feet in top shape, ready to "power walk" or ready to slip on open-toe shoes. Some of my most relaxing moments are having attention lavished on my feet.

If regular professional pedicures do not fit into your lifestyle, make an effort to give yourself a pedicure at home whenever you can. First, soak your feet in warm, sudsy water, and use a pumice stone on the bottom of your feet and toes to smooth calluses and remove dead skin. Then use a soft nail brush to scrub each toe thoroughly. I then remove my feet from the water, and using an orange stick, I gently push back the cuticle around each toe. Next, I trim and file the toenails as needed. Finally, I use a rich cream to lovingly massage my feet, taking time to give attention to each toe. I finish my home pedicure by "misting" my feet with an inexpensive skin antiseptic, which I keep in diluted form in a plastic misting bottle. The antiseptic will make your feet tingle and feel energetic and ready to go! Polish for your toes is optional. I find I usually "ruin" my toe polish, because I never have enough time to let it dry thoroughly. If you do choose to polish your toenails, all the same tips for nails given before apply to your toes as well. No chipped polish, please!

Your feet and hands are the places you can shine. They are the outward symbols of how you feel about yourself. Well-groomed, well-maintained, healthy feet and hands are the signature of confident, proud, curvy women.

"CHALLENGING" AREAS

By "challenging" areas, I mean any part of your body that may not be your favorite. Your upper arms, your hips, your thighs, your lower abs. Any part of your body that you would choose to alter (even just a little) if you could. Once you have identified the area (or areas) on which to work, I want you to begin practicing loving hands-on touch and massage on that very area. For so long, we have ignored our bodies, and especially those areas that have brought us emotional pain. By learning to touch those areas caringly, forgivingly, and openly, we can begin to repair the damaged relationship and negativity we associate with that area. You can have a hands-on session with your challenging area whenever you feel the need. It only requires a little privacy and a few quiet moments. I like to spend hands-on time with my stomach when I am in bed ready to go to sleep.

Slowly and sensuously, I begin to rub my stomach in small circular motions, first one direction and then the other. As I am rubbing, I try to notice the way my stomach feels to the touch and I put words to the feelings. It feels soft. It feels mushy. It feels warm. It feels good. I do this for however long it feels right, and complete my hands-on session by sending positive feelings and love to my stomach. I thank it for functioning properly, and being so brave in a world that celebrates the flat tummy and abs of steel. I give it credit for holding its own and, for better or worse, being my stomach. I wrap it in a "blanket" of a beautiful color of my choice, surrounding it with the color, letting the color wash through, over, and around it.

After practicing loving, hands-on rituals with your own body you will recognize a change. Not necessarily a change in the "challenging area," but rather, a change in how you *feel* about that area. Hands-on loving attention creates channels in which positive energy can flow and nurture the new relationship you have created with your own body.

The Final Touch

Make a habit of hugging yourself at least once a day. By hugging I mean literally wrapping your arms around yourself as far as they will reach, holding on tight, and squeezing. A big, soft, loving embrace from *you* to *you*. If you are so inclined (as I sometimes am), go ahead and kiss your forearms as you are hugging yourself.

Although your first reaction may be "no way, I can't do it," I encourage you to give it a try. By taking a moment to stop and physically love yourself in the body you possess, you are reinforcing the message to your own self as well as spreading the positive vibes to those around you. You will receive an extra boost when people might ask, "What are you doing?" And you can confidently respond, "Giving a hug to the person I love the most!"

In my early twenties, I went through a very lonely period. I longed for someone to hug me. Someone to love me. Someone to hold me. Someone to take care of me. Someone to adore me. I remember lying in bed crying for someone, *anyone* to hold me. As a remedy for my loneliness (as I am not one to stay sad too long if I can find ways to "fix" it), I began taking time to relax, or meditate. I taught myself to calmly, slowly, and peacefully relax, breathe, and open my mind, and my life, to new situations.

Over time and during periods of deep relaxation and

"higher learning," I heard inside of my own head the answers I had been searching for. They sounded exactly like this: "Catherine needs to hug Catherine." "Catherine needs to love Catherine." "Catherine needs to hold Catherine." "Catherine needs to take care of Catherine." "Catherine needs to adore Catherine." They came to me as clear as a bell. I had been expecting someone to love me without loving myself first. Doesn't make sense, does it? Until we can love and accept ourselves as we are, meaningful love from others is impossible.

This is how hugging myself got started. I did, and still do, many other things to love myself including the hugging. Most of these techniques you will find within the eight steps in this book! Hugging was a start. I usually do it when I have completed some finite task. Such as completing a chapter of this book. Or at the end of a particularly draining meeting. Or, most often, when I finish one of my walks. I love to walk, and when I am rounding the last corner, heading back home, I give my arms a big stretch over my head and then wrap them around my body, giving myself a big, strong hug. Sometimes I kiss my forearms and pat myself on the shoulders. I congratulate myself for a job well done, showing gratitude for a body that is big and strong and able to walk and move, and reminding myself that I am special and beautiful in my own unique, wonderful way.

Give yourself a quick hug right now. This hug signifies the successful start of a new relationship with your body! See how far we've come? Let's move ahead and take some time to focus on the "outer" steps—beginning with a complete body assessment.

1. Put your scale away, in a closet, out of sight. You are not a number on a scale and it has no bearing on your worth as a human being. If you need a "measure" for your body, use how you feel and/or the fit of your clothes.

2. Take a moment to describe your idea of a perfect relationship with your body. What sort of ideals would it be based on? How would you nurture this relationship?

3. Are you prepared to love yourself as you are right now? If so, you must recognize that there will be positive fallout and reverberations that will spring up all over your life. Are you ready to accept these positive changes? If so, copy the following sentence and post it in a place where you can read it every day:

> *I* [put your first name here] *have made the decision to begin loving myself as I am today. I will love and nurture the body I have every day from this day forward, putting to rest any preconceived ideas of what my weight should be. I will make every effort to appreciate and celebrate my body as it is today, regardless of a dress size or number on a scale, and work to keep it healthy, strong, and beautiful.*

4. Use a separate sheet and list your inner assets by completing the following sentences: "I like_____" and "I can _____." Think of as many as you can, and keep the lists handy so that you may add to them when you think of new inner assets!

5. Write all of your inner assets on little slips of paper (one per slip) and mix them up in a bowl or container. Pull one out at random and read it out loud each time you catch yourself in a negative mood or thought!

6. Practice one or more of the hands-on body pampering rituals. Concentrate on the "challenging areas" of your body, lavishing them with *more* rituals, *more* frequently.

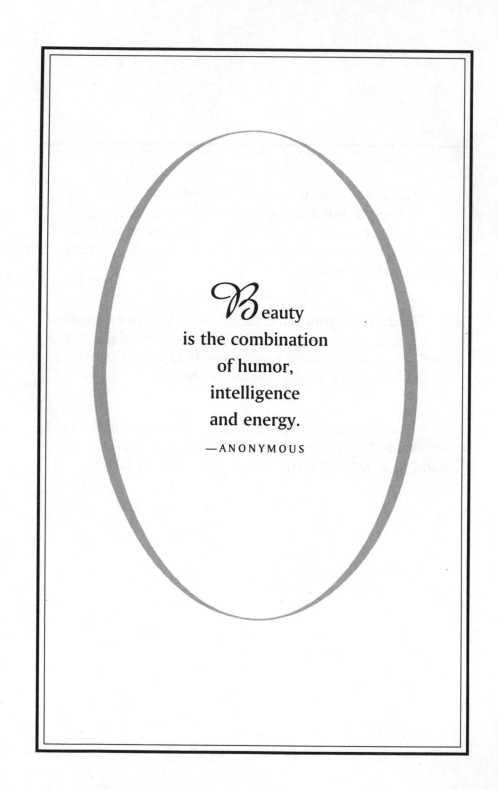

$\mathcal{B}$eauty
is the combination
of humor,
intelligence
and energy.

—ANONYMOUS

4

Assess Your Outer Strengths

*A*ll too often, we concentrate time and energy on our weaknesses instead of our strengths. We look to that which is "wrong" with our bodies before we celebrate the things that are "right." Whether we realize it or not, as we are trying to "fix" our body to fit some unrealistic ideal, our self-worth and self-esteem take a real beating. In this step, I will lead you through a total-body assessment, helping you to identify and highlight your strengths, your assets, and your selling points. Our goal in this step is to conduct a head-to-toe body survey and, in the process, identify those parts and areas we want to accentuate and celebrate—not cover, hide, fix, or change.

Whether or not you choose to believe it, we *all* have assets worthy of our attention and adornment. In Step 3 we looked at our inner assets. Now we will take a tour of your body—a personalized head-to-toe exploration of your *outer* assets—those aspects that are visible in the mirror.

Outer Assessment

Before we move to the actual exercise of conducting an *outer* assessment of our bodies—that process of taking inventory of what we see in the mirror—we need to take a moment to revisit the concept altogether.

Outer assessment is not a new idea. In fact, most

well-dressed women have learned the power of proper body assessment. They teach themselves to work well with what they have going for them, and downplay the rest. No woman I know likes every single aspect of her body. But smart women know how to draw attention to those parts of their bodies they like.

For some reason, most women of size have forgotten how to do this—how to assess themselves properly. This step will show you how to recover those assessment abilities. By participating in a personalized outer assessment, rediscovering all of our positives, we will be well on the road toward looking and feeling better about ourselves.

Retraining Your Eye

Before we begin an outer assessment with the twenty-point checklist, let's do a quick brush-up on *how* we look at ourselves in the mirror. Most women need to train their eye to see their *positives* before they notice their *negatives*. How many times have we seen women of all shapes and sizes pass a mirror and make disapproving grimaces or negative comments about the way they look? "Oh, my hair looks a mess." "This dress makes me look fat." "My thighs are huge!" "Boy, is my stomach ever sticking out!" "Why did I wear this? It looks terrible." Or, just plain and simple, "I hate the way I look." Each time we do this we are reinforcing the aspects we dislike rather than the ones we like, further ingraining a negative thought pattern. Does this make any sense? No. But it is a cycle that is difficult to break.

Positive thoughts are the building blocks for accepting ourselves the way we are—as they set the foundation for positive change. Dwelling on the negatives only reinforces them and validates them further, making them seem more real and important than they are.

This malady of only seeing the "bad and the ugly" is especially prevalent in women of size. We have been trained to dwell on our *"bad"* body parts . . . the *"big"* parts . . . the parts that make us look different from the fashion models we see in the magazines. We are taught to hold ourselves up in comparison to thin women—although it may be an ideal that we can never achieve. Television, magazines, and the movies show us what they think we *should* look like. All the "shoulds" become very depressing after a while, and we give up on the concept of a positive body image altogether. It's too much pressure to try to live up to.

The pressure can be overwhelming to the point of emotional paralysis. I notice that women (of all sizes) often have pictures of models from the fashion magazines pasted on their refrigerator doors, supposedly discouraging them from eating. I have never known a case where this has actually had some positive impact. In fact, I think it only creates frustration while reinforcing an unrealistic image in their minds. Inspirational refrigerator "art" is fine, but I encourage women to pick something *truly* inspirational. Instead of vapid Supermodel X in a string bikini, I have my own versions of visual inspiration—a photo of Ella Fitzgerald—dressed to the nines, sassy and fabulous; a postcard of an old Steichen photo of Greta Garbo looking pensive and chic; a hauntingly beautiful photo of Jessye Norman (world-famous opera diva) in profile, and a postcard of a Matisse reclining nude (well rounded, naturally!). These images lift my spirits, encouraging me to celebrate my own positives instead of berating myself for not looking like a supermodel.

Believe it or not, we can actually learn something important from *men* in this area. Men traditionally and instinctively *downplay their shortcomings* and *boast about their assets*. Most balding men will never call attention to their baldness, but rather draw attention to their well-defined biceps, or yesterday's excellent golf score. If a man is large, you certainly won't hear him complaining about his corpulent rear end. Instead he'll be telling you about his high-powered job or how he's planning to take sky-diving lessons.

Men are really very good at this. It pervades almost every area of their lives. When given the choice, men generally choose to build themselves up, rather than beat themselves down. Have you noticed this? "I don't need a map, I know how to get there." "No problem, I can install that air-conditioning unit." "Let me program the VCR." Same idea. Men *boast* instead of *berate* in many areas of their lives. Perhaps they experience the same body-image doubts and insecurities as women, but they generally *downplay* them, focusing on their positives instead.

Remembering how to see the positives first takes just a little concentrated time and effort and a bit of assistance to get you started. Through practice, patience, and a willingness to accept a positive outlook for your life, you will *only* be seeing the beautiful, unique qualities you possess. I will assist you in conducting your own body assessment, and together, as a united force of beautiful, well-rounded women, we will teach the rest of womankind how to look in a mirror and immediately say something *positive* rather than negative.

Women of size all over the world should be paying themselves compliments, admiring their bodies, celebrating their strengths, and reinforcing aspects about themselves that they love. Imagine how wonderful it is to look in the mirror and see your positives *first*!

No More Lumping

I've found that the biggest hurdle we have to overcome is to avoid what I call "lumping." Lumping means seeing oneself as one big lump instead of various and assorted parts. Women of size tend to lump all their body parts together when they look in the mirror. They only glance quickly at their reflection, and give themselves one quick, generalized label—*fat*. Without differentiating or defining the separate elements that make up our bodies, we further alienate ourselves from our bodies, and choose only to see a lump.

Instead, like scientists, we need to go over the body bit by bit, top to bottom and bottom to top, discovering that we are much more than an amorphous lump. We need to study our bodies and notice that we *all* have a shape, a structure—and that we *all* have parts of our body we like. Parts that have been ignored over time, "lumped" and forgotten. No matter what we weigh, we are the sum of our different and unique parts—some great, some just okay, and some that we choose to downplay. Our bodies are *not* lumps but rather, a beautiful and varied collection of these parts which work together to create a single, unique work of art—you! We can choose to work on certain aspects accentuating or downplaying them to our desire—celebrating our unique form.

"You Have Such a Pretty Face"

These six words are among the *most* detrimental one could ever utter to a well-rounded woman. I know you have heard them as many times as I have. Do you feel the same way? It took me many years to come to some resolution in my own mind as to why a "compliment" could make me so angry. Although the person who says to you "you have such a pretty face" believes he or she is paying a compliment, it is actually a backhanded criticism about our weight.

Those words would incite more and more anger each time they were said to me, and yet, I would force myself to say thank you when what I really wanted to say was "!#*$&^@* you"! "But, darling, you have such a pretty face" does not mean that the person believes my face is pretty. The actual translation of this statement is something much closer to: "I don't approve or accept the size of your body," or, "You would be pretty except for the fact that you are fat." It is another way of saying, "You don't fit into my idea of beauty, and because of that, I will not acknowledge you from the neck down" (yes, the old neck up syndrome again!)

Once I grasped what was being implied in that statement, I was able to account for my anger and frustration and decide how I was going to react the next time it was said to me. Once I realized *all* the beautiful parts of my body (not just my face), I began to answer like this: "Thank you. *And* I have a great body. I've got fabulous legs and dynamite curves. Want to see?" This may sound outrageous at first, but after I had accurately assessed my positives, I was armed with a frank, honest comeback. I had the complete confidence to talk openly with others about the wonderful parts of my body in addition to "my pretty face." By exuding confidence in our assets, we are then able to assist others in recognizing our bountiful beauty below the neck!

Mirror, Mirror, You Are My Friend

Acknowledging your below-the-neck beauty begins by making friends with the mirror. Many women are terrified of mirrors, attaching to them wildly unrealistic and warped images of themselves. The more out of touch we become with our bodies, the less and less frequently we look in a mirror. If we do glance at our reflection, it is only for fleeting moments, blurring our vision or only looking at ourselves from the neck up. The fact of the matter is that women of size are afraid of the key tool to assessment: the mirror.

Mirrors only reflected the pain I felt about my body. Everytime I even glanced in a mirror I would be overcome by feelings of inadequacy and shame. When my self-esteem was low, I despised mirrors . . . dodged them, ditched them, and avoided them like the plague. Not until I began modeling did I learn how to make friends with the mirror.

Instead of seeing the mirror as my enemy, I decided to think of it as a member of my team—part of the cohesive force working toward my improved well-being. This did not happen overnight. It happened slowly. Little by little, I started to focus on different areas of my body— culling the positives and learning to downplay the rest, all the while overcoming my fears of facing the mirror. The more I looked, the more positives I found. The more positives I discovered, the more I became increasingly confident about my relationship with the mirror, and it became an integral part of my everyday life. The mirror became my comrade rather than my foe, and I learned to use it as a tool for self-esteem, not a weapon for self-hatred.

The mirror is the primary tool we need in order to take stock of what we have to work with. The best way to reacquaint yourself with your mirror is to locate all the mirrors in your house. Do you even know where they are? Do you have a full-length mirror? Is it accessible—meaning, can you see your entire image in it without any obstructions blocking your view? Go and take a look. You might be surprised to find that you do not have an unobstructed, full-length mirror. When I first searched my house I didn't. I realized that every mirror in my house made me visible only from the neck up or the waist up.

It is essential that you have a full-length mirror to begin the assessment of your body. If you discover that you do not have one, *please* go buy one. Mirrors are inexpensive and will prove to be invaluable in your assessment process. In fact, even if you *do* have one, I would suggest purchasing another. This new mirror represents your new start, a new way of looking at your body, and an affirmation of how much you love yourself. Install your new full-length mirror in a special place where you can see your body fully with the option of privacy if you choose. This new mirror belongs to you. It is your new friend and your new partner in creating a healthy relationship with your body.

Once you have found (or purchased) your full-length mirror and installed it in a accessible location, you are prepared to begin your own body assessment. You don't have to do this alone. I will guide you through the process. Additionally, you will find a Body-Positive Checklist at the end of this step to help you get started.

By the way, it is *completely* natural if you are feeling apprehensive about this process right now. After all, it has been awhile since you spent some time with the mirror, studying your own body. Allow yourself to feel the way you do right now—whether it is nervous, scared, angry or sad. You need to experience these feelings fully in order to let them pass. Feel the way they feel, acknowledge that they exist, and then concentrate on moving *through* them. Once your feelings have surfaced, there will be more space available for you to experience a multitude of new and wonderful sensations about your own body.

When you are in front of your mirror ready to assess, be sure you are wearing comfortable clothing that will allow you to move, lift, turn, and examine each area of your body. Since you might be nervous about approaching the mirror for the first time, take it slowly. Do a little bit at a time. Divide your body into "quarters" and assess only a quarter per day or even a quarter per week. There is no rush. You have the rest of your life to assess and reassess yourself.

To help you in your quest for your assets, read about each of the twenty body "points" in the following section. These are the twenty checkpoints that I use when I work one on one with women in body assessment—the backbone of outer assessments. Please note that there are infinitely *more* than twenty potential "positive aspects" of our bodies. Add as many as you wish based on your own body discoveries. I am sharing these with you only to get you started.

Twenty-Point Body-Positive Map

The following is a quick rundown of the twenty checkpoints I use in actual body assessments. Use them as guideposts for your own body discovery. Hopefully they will spark ideas and lead you to finding new "positives" in your own body assessment. In the Toolbox at the end of this step, you will find a copy of the Body-Positive Checklist that I use with my clients. If you wish, you can turn to it and follow along, studying your own body in the mirror and filling in the appropriate spaces. Remember, there is beauty everywhere. Train your eye to seek it out and showcase it in the best way possible.

BODY POINT 1: HAIR

How do you like your hair? Is it thick and straight or fine and wavy? Thick and wavy or fine and straight? Do you like the style and color of your hair? Do people compliment you on your haircut? Does it properly frame your face? Is it something you are proud of and take great care to maintain? There is great variation in types of lovely hair. Yours may be long or short. Heavy or light. Feel the texture. How does it feel to your touch? Soft? Smooth? Coarse? How does it feel to others when they touch it? Do you let others brush your hair? Hair, unlike other body parts we will be covering, can be an asset for most women with the correct attention and care. Loving your hair means keeping your head and scalp in healthy condition, and choosing a hair style (and perhaps color) that is flattering and well suited to your lifestyle.

Cuts and styles differ widely from person to person. So the best advice I can give is to find a stylist who you like and respect. Some questions to ask yourself about the person you choose to do your hair: "Do I feel comfortable talking to this person?" "Will he/she listen to what I want?" "Is he/she willing and able to offer suggestions/advice?" "Do I like the hairstyles he/she has given to other women?" The best way to answer most of these questions is to set up an appointment for a consultation. Most salons are quite accustomed to this practice, setting aside ten or fifteen minutes for a free chat with the opera-tor of your choice. Use the consultation to ask as many questions as you like, talking openly about what you ex-pect and telling the stylist exactly how much time you are able to spend on your hair every day. An honest, well-planned ten-minute discussion with your hair stylist *be-fore* you cut or color can save months of heartache and despair resulting from a bad cut, color, or style.

As we all know, the best part about having your hair done at a salon is having someone wash your hair. This is the type of intimate, body-positive ritual that you can replicate at home for yourself. Think of that wonderful scene in the movie *Out of Africa* when Robert Redford washes Meryl Streep's hair by the river. A wonderful scalp massage (even if it's not given by Robert Redford) can be the ultimate loving ritual for your hair and head. I eagerly await those five minutes with my head thrown back in the basin and someone washing my hair. Do you have a favorite hair washer at your salon? If so, be sure to give him/her an extra nice tip with sincere thanks and many compliments. This will ensure that they remember you the next time you are in, and maybe those five min-utes will stretch to seven, eight, or ten!

Here's a helpful tip for all of us well-rounded salon-goers. I carry my own smock to beauty salons whenever I go to have my hair cut or colored. Nothing is more annoying or demeaning than arriving for a session of hair pampering and realizing in the changing room that the smock is too small! Has this happened to you too? After living through this inconvenience one too many times, I decided to take control of the situation. I had a smock made to fit my body and I take it along whenever I have my hair done. I know it will fit and thus I avoid the changing room anxiety.

Day-to-day maintenance for your hair is based around keeping it clean, shiny, and healthy. Use a shampoo of *your* choice. *Refuse* to settle for "whatever's in the shower." Grape-scented shampoo with cartoon characters on the bottle is fine for the kids, and I know your husband needs to use the dandruff shampoo prescribed by his dermatologist, but you should insist on having your own special hair products, for your own special hair.

Every month or so, I give my hair a special conditioning treatment. I usually do this in the evening when I have a little extra time (mornings are just too rushed). I give my hair a quick wash and apply any of the small conditioning packs available in drug and cosmetic stores. I then slip into a robe and wrap my gooey, wet head in a towel. I let my hair "cook" in the towel for at least one hour, while I read, clean, sew, rest, talk on the phone, or watch television.

After removing the towel, I thoroughly rinse the conditioner out of my hair and dry, set, or style as usual. These monthly treatments help to keep hair soft and shiny, especially if you are hard on your hair as I am—always using hot rollers, hair dryers, or having your hair professionally (chemically) treated with highlights, color or permanents.

I find that many well-rounded women have beautiful hair—well nourished and healthy. We take in enough calories and nutrients to stimulate and maintain gorgeous, healthy hair and scalps! Hair can be an asset for all lovely, large ladies!

BODY POINT 2: EYES

What color are they? How long as it been since you really looked into your own eyes? What do you see? Green emeralds? Blue aquamarines? Amber-colored jewels with flecks of gold? Are your eyes exotically almond shaped? Would you describe your eyes as sparkling? Expressive? Are your eyes the true mirror of your soul? Take a moment to look deeply and passionately into your own eyes. Are you properly showcasing your eyes with graceful, clean, arching eyebrows? Do you accentuate their color with subtle, natural eye makeup?

If you feel you could learn how to better highlight your eyes with makeup, I would suggest seeking a professional makeup consultation. Most large department stores offer "makeovers" at their cosmetic counters. First, be a spectator, watching the different makeup artists work on different customers. Choose the one who you feel creates the most attractive, natural look (it really doesn't matter which cosmetics line they represent, as most companies produce a wide selection of colors and shades to choose from). Once you have learned how to best showcase your eyes, take a moment to acknowledge their beauty. Beauty is not only in the eye of the beholder, it's also in the eyes themselves!

BODY POINT 3: LIPS/MOUTH

Your lips and mouth, including your teeth, are one of the most sensuous areas of your body. Study your lips. Are they full and rounded? Pouty? Heart-shaped? Believe it or not, these days women pay thousands of dollars for lip implants—an attempt to create fuller, more sensuous lips, an asset many well-rounded women already have! Rounded, fleshy, fuller lips look especially fabulous on the plus-size woman. Our lips represent the fullness with which we choose to live our lives . . . full of kissing, full of tasting and drinking life, things our smaller sisters are sometimes afraid to do!

No matter what shape your mouth is, there are ways to accentuate and highlight the beauty. Lipstick is a must, unless you are one of the *very* few lucky people whose lips are naturally cherry colored. You can enjoy many different shades of lipstick depending on your mood, the season, or what you are wearing. I do suggest, however, that you have one favorite, a permanent standby, a trusty shade that you know will look great no matter what. It will be different for each person.

I once heard a Frenchwoman describe how she likes her mouth to look. She says, "I put on my lipstick—a deep, deep red—and then roughly and vigorously rub it all off with a tissue. I then reapply it—but just a little— giving my lips color and a 'bruised look'—as if they had been bruised from kissing all night long."

Every woman can have a beautiful mouth if she re- members just two things. First, always try to use your mouth to say loving and positive things about yourself and others. And second, always smile. Smile frequently and with abandon. Smiling releases certain face muscles, creating a more relaxed and attractive facial expression. Frowning actually takes more work than smiling. Practice smiling as much as you can. Find new occasions to smile. I read somewhere that if you are faced with having to make a particularly difficult phone call, try smiling the whole time you are talking. It changes the timbre of your voice and transfers the positive vibrations to the other party. Smiling is the easiest way to show off your beautiful mouth, feel instantly better about yourself, and make everyone around you feel better.

BODY PART 4: NOSE

Have you ever studied your nose? Is it an asset to your body? What's its shape and size? Is it small, big, pug, Roman, elegant, aristocratic, unusual? How does your nose complement your face? I don't believe that there is such a thing as a "bad" nose. In fact, I have a difficult time understanding why people choose to have a "nose job" for cosmetic reasons. Elective cosmetic surgery can be an esteem booster if it is done for the right reasons. But when it comes to noses, I just love the fact that everyone's nose is so *unique*.

The best way to study your nose and discover its shape is by looking at your profile. Try using two hand-held mirrors to see your nose in profile. Or have someone take a Polaroid photograph of your face in profile. It is only in profile that we can study the shape of our own nose and appreciate its sculptural value for our face. I believe in wearing your nose proudly, displaying it as you would a family crest or coat of arms.

BODY PART 5: EARS

Ears are a very sensuous and distinctive part of your body. Do you traditionally choose to draw attention toward your ears or away from them? A good way to tell is to take note whether or not you wear your hair covering or exposing your ears. Do you wear earrings to adorn and accentuate your ears? Pierced or unpierced, you should know what type of earring looks best on you. Do you look better in big, gold, Gypsyesque hoops or simple pearl or diamond studs? (See Step 6 for hints on how to gauge the correct size and scale for your accessories, including earrings.)

Like shells adorning the sides of your face, your ears are a very sensitive and sensual area of the body. Decide if you like your ears and if so, pull your hair back away from your face, unveiling them for the world to see.

BODY PART 6: NECK

Necks can be so beautiful. The gentle slope that leads from the head to the torso is both inviting and mysterious. Arching one's neck opens it for a kiss, a nuzzle, or a caress. The neck holds mysteries, as it is the portal to the rest of the body—the gateway that connects the mind and the body. It is a passageway encasing vital pipelines for life. I feel things more sensitively on my neck, especially the back of my neck. Do you?

In studying your own neck in the mirror, notice if it is suitable for adornment. It may not be. Sometimes even the most beautiful necklace cannot match the beauty of the unadorned, naked neck. Are you interrupting the perfect vertical line of your neck by wearing a necklace that hits at an unbecoming point? I believe the rule of thumb here is to either wear a very long necklace (thirty inches or longer) or a choker style (assuming your neck is long enough to do so), ruling out any necklace at a choppy mid-length (anywhere between eighteen and thirty inches). (More on this in Step 6.) Experiment first, and try a variety of lengths to see which suits your neck the best. Choose clothing with necklines that showcase your beautiful neck. And regardless if you think your neck is one of your assets or not, always remember to dab perfume at your neckline—especially at the base of your neck. Anatomically speaking, body heat is centralized at your jugular vein (in your neck), and perfume is warmed and disseminated most quickly from this area.

BODY PART 7: SHOULDERS

Your shoulders have the responsibility of carrying your body forward into the world effortlessly and joyfully. It's no coincidence that Atlas used his shoulders to carry the globe, as they are a pivotal point of strength for our body. Our shoulders are a balance beam, holding all other parts in alignment and creating a strong horizontal plane from which the torso can "hang." Are you holding your shoulders strong, tall, and straight in line with your back? Shoulders assist in keeping your body erect and aligned. Standing up straight, holding your shoulders down away from your ears, creates a strong body silhouette, elongating and balancing your body frame.

When you look at your shoulders in the mirror, are they square, broad, and flat, or more rounded, narrow, and curved? If you have big square shoulders you may decide that shoulder pads are overkill, and only make you look like a linebacker. I regularly remove all shoulder pads from clothes I buy (or model), knowing that my broad shoulders do not need the extra padding. If you do not have especially broad shoulders, however, you will want to figure out the best type of shoulder pad and use it with everything you own. Many women make the mistake of accepting and using the pads that are attached in articles of clothing they buy. Try different shoulder pad shapes and sizes and don't be afraid to rip a pair out of a garment you own and replace them with something better.

With a careful analysis of your shoulders, and the

determination of whether or not to enhance with pads, your shoulders have the potential of becoming a valued asset. Once you have created a beautiful horizontal line at shoulder level, accentuating your own God-given shoulders, you have set in place the framework for the rest of your body.

BODY PART 8: ARMS

Don't panic. I promise I won't force you into wearing sleeveless blouses, unless you feel comfortable doing so. I hear so many complaints from the women I work with about their upper arms—and about 50 percent of them are valid complaints. The rest are vain attempts to live up to an unrealistic ideal of what arms "should" look like. In fact, I once heard a silly girl I know (a size 10) say that she wouldn't ever lift anything heavy, because she feared developing muscles and only wanted "skinny, little bony arms." Ha! Unless you are genetically predisposed to have the arms of an eight-year old (and she wasn't), it isn't going to happen. Fleshiness does not have to be un-attractive. I simply ask you now to take a good, long look at your upper arms in the mirror and give them a fair assessment.

As you study your arms, think of all your strong muscles that live underneath the skin. Flex your muscles in front of the mirror and see what they look like. You might be surprised to find definition you didn't know was there. Simple day-to-day chores and tasks can help to create and maintain muscle tone in your biceps and triceps without your ever setting foot in a gym or weight room. Carrying groceries, lifting your children, opening and shutting the garage door, raking leaves, and sweeping or vacuuming are all activities that can lead to strong, firm upper-arm muscle tone.

Enough about the muscle; how about the skin? Take a moment to feel the skin on your upper arms. Feel all around—on top *and* underneath. Upper-arm skin is usually softer than skin elsewhere, because we take such great pains to cover it up. As a result it is protected against the elements and remains soft.

Appreciate the soft skin and at least pose the question to yourself: "Can I consider my upper arms an asset?" If the answer is "yes" or even "maybe"—terrific! Celebrate by remembering to moisturize regularly, keeping the tender skin soft to the touch, and by not being so afraid to take off your jacket to show some upper arm! If, after reading this and doing a careful analysis of your upper arms, you decide they are not one of your positives, so be it. I will not make you take off your jacket. Just remember to use your upper arms to embrace yourself regularly . . . telling yourself how much you love and accept each part of your body. Use your arms to hug and embrace others as well. Although you may not consider your upper arms one of your assets, those who receive your embraces might treasure their strength and softness.

The length between your elbow and your wrist comprises your lower arm. Study carefully this angular extremity of your body. Notice its shape. Is it rounded or flat? Make a first, and see what it does to the muscles in your arm. Watch the muscles tighten and release as you clench and unclench your fist.

Have you ever acknowledged how much grace and fluidity of movement can be read through the forearms? Belly dancers, hula dancers, and ballet dancers exemplify how amazingly beautiful the lower arms can be. Dancers really know how to use the elegant extremity—

stretching, reaching, and worshiping every move their arms make. Models, too, know the secret elegance of arms. Look at photographs in fashion magazines and examine how the models use their lower arms to express emotion. They turn, contort, study, and elongate their arms to create a look or mood.

Notice the skin and hair on your forearms. Are there freckles? A beauty mark? Is the hair blond or dark? See how smooth your arms feel as you use your hands to stroke them? Do you choose to adorn your wrists with bracelets? Do the bracelets help to create a clean, elongated line? Conceptually, I like the idea of cuff bracelets because they invoke images of strength and power. However, I believe that on fuller figures, they tend to break the line between elbow and wrist, creating an unattractive, chopped-up look. Your arms are the exclamation points of your body. Practice moving and floating them around in front of the mirror. Learn how they can become the perfect punctuation for your life.

BODY PART 9: HANDS

How do you feel about your hands? When you are studying yourself in your mirror, hold your hands up and really take a good look at them. I know we all lead busy lives, but taking care of our hands is one of those telltale signs that indicate how much time and effort we spend on our upkeep.

When's the last time someone complimented you on your hands? Do you like the way they look right now as you study them in the mirror? As you are looking at their reflection in the mirror, blur your vision a little and concentrate only on their shape. Don't focus on the nails, but rather the size and scale of your hands and fingers.

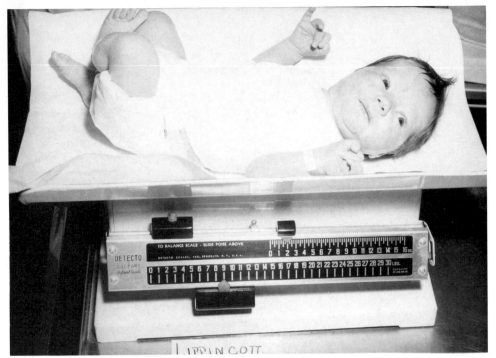

One day old. The first of many weigh-ins. At nine pounds two ounces, I was a big, healthy baby. Photo courtesy of The Lippincott Family.

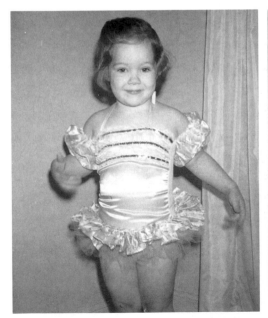

Age 2½. A well-rounded dancer is a beautiful dancer.
Photo courtesy of The Lippincott Family.

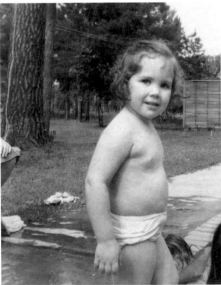

Age 3. Topless with no tummy shame. It took years to get back to this mind-set. Photo courtesy of The Lippincott Family.

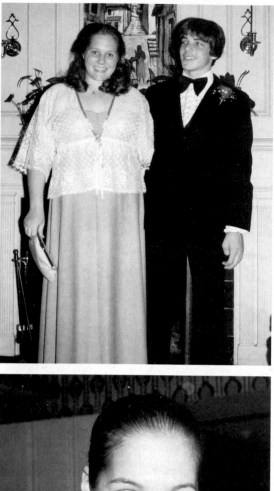

Age 15. A dress that fit. It was difficult to find "formal" dresses in larger sizes that didn't look too matronly. This one was from Lane Bryant as I recall. Photo courtesy of The Lippincott Family.

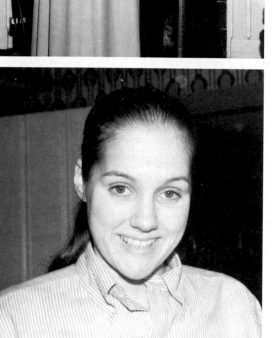

Age 18. The closest I've come to a mug shot. Check-in photo at a well-known weight reduction camp in North Carolina. Not a happy camper. I remember that I was feeling sad and lost and depressed about having to go on yet another diet. Photo courtesy of Catherine Lippincott.

Age 17. After five months on a medically supervised fast. I am finally thin, but sacrificed my health to get there. I lost 100 pounds, and gained it all back in less time than it took me to lose it. Photo courtesy of The Lippincott Family.

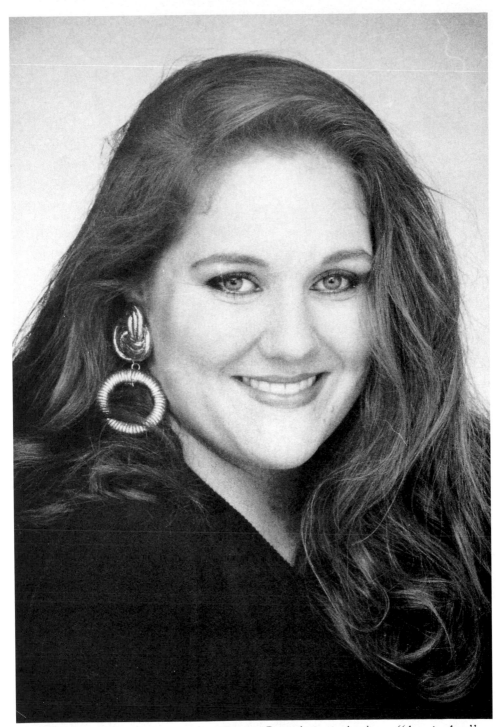

Age 21. My first year in New York and the first "head shot" ever taken of me for modeling. I was a size 24, actually not a great size for modeling, but it was one of my first small steps toward accepting my body. Photo by Elaine Velaochaga.

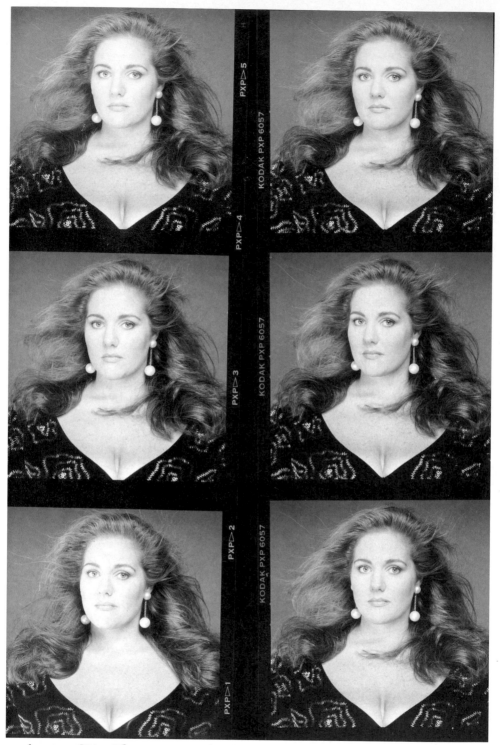

Age 24. My <u>Cosmo</u> cover look. A high glam test shoot. By this time I had done several small modeling jobs in New York and my confidence was growing. Photos by Joe Chaves.

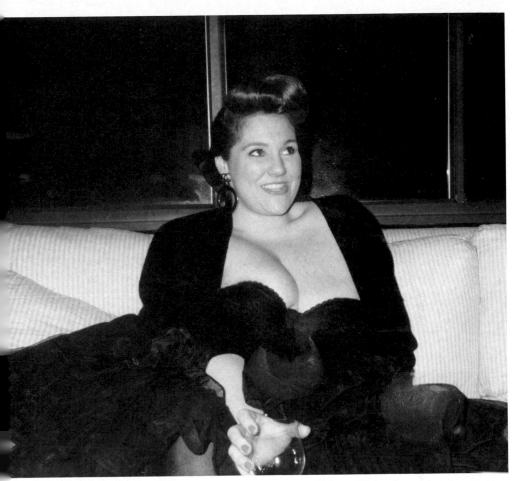

Age 25. (Over?) working my assets. New York party days.
A size 22 who is slowly figuring out that glamour doesn't stop at
a size 8. Photo by Billy B.

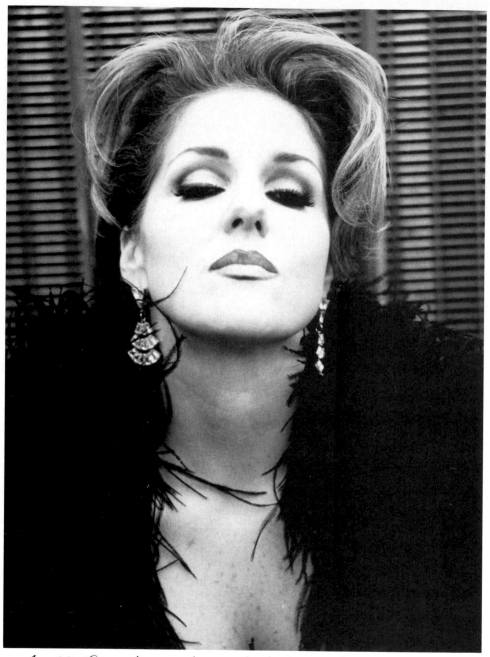

Age 29. Over-the-top glamour look shot on the streets of New York. Photo by Michelle McCabe.

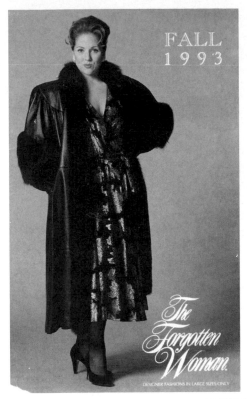

FALL
1993

The Forgotten Woman.

DESIGNER FASHIONS IN LARGE SIZES ONLY

Age 30. A national catalogue cover—at last! Photo courtesy of "The Forgotten Woman." 1–800–TFW–1424.

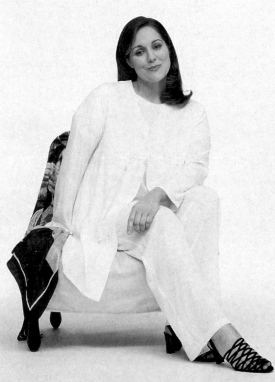

Age 32. A clean and simple '90s catalogue look. Photo courtesy of "Ulla Popken" New Classics in sizes 12 and up. 1–800–245–8552 (ULLA).

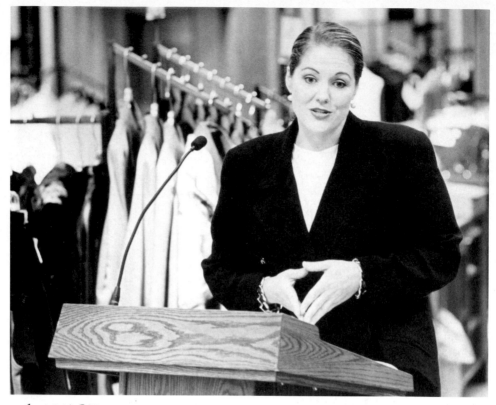

*Age 33. Me in action—
sharing the Well
Rounded message with
women of size in
department stores around
the country.* Photo courtesy of
Catherine Lippincott.

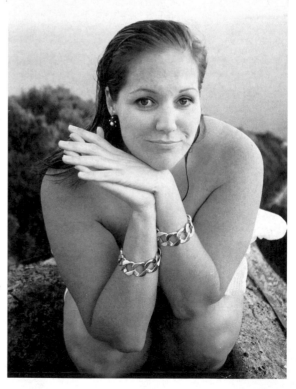

*Age 33. Me. No
makeup. Happy.* Photo by
Richard Buckley.

Do the rings you wear flatter the size of your hands? Stretch each of your fingers, as piano players often do when warming up. Bend and straighten, flex and relax— send thunderbolts of positive energy from each of your ten fingertips.

Think of all the tasks your hands do each day. Your hands hold, carry, and clasp things. Your hands hold the food that you are preparing to feed your family, they carry your books to and from school, they clasp the pen that signs the contract and business agreements that provide your income. Your hands make your life happen. Even if you don't think of your hands as one of your favorite body parts, your hands deserve recognition for all that they do.

BODY PART 10: BACK

It won't be easy to get a good look at your back, but I want you to try. Use two mirrors—one hand-held and the other full-length, or both full-length if you have them. Begin to notice details about your back. Maybe this is the first time you have taken a close look at it. Does it look smooth? Freckled? Soft? Firm? Can you see your shoulder blades and back muscles move as your turn and twist? Now that you are having a good look, do you think you would you feel comfortable wearing clothes that show off some or all of your back? I have a very simple, oversized black cotton V-neck sweater, which I wear *backward* with the V in the back. Showing some of your back is a nice alternative to showing front cleavage. And it always makes for great exits!

Your back is beautiful. It is beautiful because of the service it performs. It supports you with strength, power, and grace. Use your back to stand tall, be counted, and face the world with a strong, confident posture.

BODY PART 11: CHEST

Chests or "bosoms" have been a topic of interest (and sometimes awe) for centuries. Think of all the attention the bosom has received. Breast reductions or breast enlargements are commonplace these days. The bra has flourished over the years. You have choices such as minimizers, padded, push-ups, demis, or even a bra just for sports activities. The days of binding the breasts or burning bras are long over.

There is no one standard size chest for well-rounded women. You could be flat-chested, well-endowed, or somewhere in between. There is a wide range of size and shapes of breasts. Most savvy women decide how to create a flattering silhouette of the bust by acknowledging what they have to work with and addressing it properly. Some choose to show it off, some don't.

The bosom may or may not be an area of the body we wish to accentuate. It's obviously a very personal decision. I have one girlfriend who is very well endowed, and she does everything she can to cover up her chest. All her clothes conceal rather than reveal. On the other hand, I have another friend who considers her bosom to be an asset, and chooses clothing that accentuate her chest. Some women are self-conscious about being flat-chested and others revel in the fact that they are absolved from always having to wear a bra. Again, it's a personal issue and one that you have choices about how to handle!

Give yourself a good look in the mirror and take a moment to study your chest. How do you describe your own chest? Are you more likely to conceal or reveal? Do you tend to wear a more revealing V or scoop neckline or a less revealing jewel (rounded) neck? Do you wear bras or undergarments that are well constructed and properly fitted? Over the years, having been in hundreds of dressing rooms with hundreds of women, I have noticed that by and large women are not wearing the correct bra or foundation garment for their bodies.

No matter if you want to accentuate or downplay your bosom, the right foundation is essential to looking great (and feeling great too!). Please invest the time and money to be properly "fitted" for your bras and foundation garments. Most large department stores offer this service for free. You will notice an immediate change in the mirror when you are properly supported by the right bra.

Your chest is not just your bosom. Your chest includes the strong muscles that support the bosom and upper torso. Take a couple of deep breaths and watch your chest expand and contract. Think of the protection, balance, and security your chest provides.

BODY PART 12: WAIST

The question you want to ask yourself here as you look at yourself in the mirror is *Do I have the delineation of a waist?* Rest assured that there is absolutely no "right" or "wrong" answer to this question. Some women have a defined waist and others do not. It all depends on our body shape.

Generally speaking, women of size have four different body "silhouettes"—according to Frances Leto Zangrillo, the associate professor of fashion design and apparel for the Fashion Institute of Technology in New York. In his textbook, *Fashion Design for the Plus-Size*, he

121

defines each of the four shapes as the rectangular-8 shape, the pear shape, the barrel shape, and the box shape.

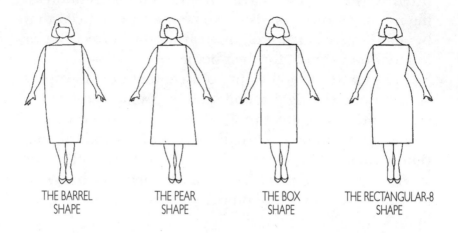

THE BARREL SHAPE   THE PEAR SHAPE   THE BOX SHAPE   THE RECTANGULAR-8 SHAPE

No one body type is "right" or "better" than any other. I introduce these shapes only so that they may help you to recognize if your body has a defined waist or not. Generally speaking, the "barrel" shape and the "box" shape tend *not* to have definition at the waist, whereas the "rectangular-8" shape and the "pear" shape *do* have some definition at the waist. Can you identify loosely which shape your body most resembles?

Obviously, there are ways to dress stylishly and comfortably for *all* body types. Women with some waist definition might feel comfortable wearing pants with a fitted waist, whereas an A-line dress might be a better option for women with little or no waist definition. Your waist can be an asset regardless of your body type. All it takes is for you to lovingly acknowledge, accept, and celebrate your own natural, flexible waist—*where*ever or *how*ever it hits the line of your body!

BODY PART 13: LOWER BELLY/ABS

Let's agree to make Body Part 13 lucky number 13 for *every*body! Whether we like or dislike our lower abdominals, it's essential to make an effort to surround them with positive supportive energy. Of all the body parts, this is the one area *I* need to spend the most time accepting and loving. How about you? Do you like your abs and lower belly? Or just tolerate them?

Bellies are tough. For a woman, so much goes on down there. To begin with, women are born with more fatty tissue in the lower belly. Nature pads us more than men so we can carry and nourish babies, surrounding them with an extra layer of "cushion" for protection. As a result, women are generally fleshier in the area surrounding her reproductive organs.

I work continually on loving my lower belly. I try to do movements and activities that stretch and strengthen the muscles *underneath*. Whether you realize it or not, the strong abdominal muscles buried deep under the surface of your belly are the ones that are connected with supporting the lower back. I try to touch my lower belly when I can, gently massaging it in small circles, eliminating all negative thoughts associated with this body area. I draw on positive images of the belly, thinking about the happy, wise, and benevolent Buddha, whose belly brings good luck to those who lovingly rub it!

BODY PARTS 14, 15, AND 16: HIPS/DERRIERE/THIGHS

I group these body parts together for two reasons. First of all, body parts 14, 15, and 16 are the three real "lulus" I hear the most complaints about. The hips, derriere, and thighs can be real self-esteem busters for many women. Secondly, this entire area of the body on *all* women has been biologically and genetically predisposed to store fat.

Again, like the lower belly, nature decided that this region is where women, the childbearers, will store the extra fatty tissue needed for child carrying, childbearing, and nursing—activities that require more calories than normal. It is here that the preservation of the species is ensured with storage of fat in case of lean days, lean months, or lean years, as our forefathers and foremothers had to endure. Pretty serious stuff. Be forewarned: if you try to mess with Mother Nature, you probably won't win.

Hips (not to be confused with the *derriere*) are those feminine protrusions that create the bottom curve when we draw a curvy figure eight. Hips show up in a front-on (or rear-on) view of our bodies. You don't see your hip shape from a profile. Your *derriere* (bottom, rear end) can be seen only from the back. Try using the two-mirror technique to get a good vantage on your posterior assets. Your *thighs* are your upper legs—sides, front, and back. Okay. Now that we have located each, let's talk about them.

Form follows function, and nowhere is this more apparent than in the lower regions of the female body. Women are meant to have hips, butts, and thighs as part of the physiology of being the baby machine. In fact, your hipbones actually expand outward (ouch) when you are pregnant to accommodate the size of the baby. Altogether, this baby-bearing region is a completely perfect, well-oiled, efficient machine. Of course I don't have to remind you that the ancient images of the fertility goddesses all have well-endowed hips, rear, and thighs to celebrate and draw attention to the uniqueness of the female form.

Additionally, women move and sway these three areas of the body (especially the hips and derriere) in ways that men cannot. Like it or not, these are the va-va-va-voom parts of a woman. The inherently feminine ability to "shake" one's hips, or to walk with the hips gently swaying from side to side, is said to originate in the animal kingdom where the swaying and sashaying of the lower torso acts to attract the "attention" of the male animal, thus assisting in the preservation of the species. I don't know if that translates directly into modern human behavior, but suffice it to say that the shape, size, and motion of our lower body is something that marks us as female; it's part of our *physiological* and *genetic* makeup.

Now that you have been reminded of some of our biological history, perhaps we can learn to appreciate our lower bodies and the unique function they serve. This is what I ask of you. Take a good look; feel, touch, and move your lower body—hips, butt, and thighs. Sway the whole package a bit from side to side. Notice how it glides and moves effortlessly with a natural rhythm and flow. Are you mistakenly hiding a part of your body that could be celebrated for its natural shape and curve? Evaluate whether you would feel comfortable wearing a well-fitted garment that accentuates your hips, bottom, and thighs.

For this general area of the body, including the hips, derriere, and thighs, I will not ask you to flaunt them or to wear butt-clinging fabrics. I also won't recommend thigh creams or magic cellulite-removing kits. What I will ask you to do is to honestly and intellectually approach this area of your body with understanding, respect, and approval.

If you are shying away from this topic altogether, then you are likely to be one who will chose to *downplay* these body parts. There is no harm in this whatsoever as long as downplaying doesn't turn into denigration or loathing of this female attribute. No matter what their size or shape, concentrate on squaring your hips to face the future. Use these strong, fleshy, inherently feminine qualities to move ahead with power, confidence, acceptance, and love.

BODY PART 17: KNEES

Our knees are a flexible and essential part of our anatomy—the central axis from which our legs move. Look closely at your knees in the mirror and decide if they are one of your positives. Raise and lower a skirt above and below the line of your knee. Try to recognize which is more flattering to the line of your body. Even if you wear your skirts below the knee, this doesn't mean your knees won't show. Whenever you sit, stand, bend, stretch, or dance, your knees will appear!

As women of size we should take extra special care of our knees because they assist in carrying the weight of our body. The kneecap is fairly exposed and is usually hit the hardest when we fall. (Remember all those scraped knees as a kid?) Try to avoid sitting or exercising in such a way that all of the body weight is resting on your knees, as when you are kneeling. This only creates excess stress on the knee and kneecap. Take time occasionally to gently massage the kneecap and its surrounding muscles, remembering the toll they take for us every day.

BODY PART 18: LOWER LEGS/CALVES

I believe that well-rounded women have great legs, especially great lower legs and calves. My theory is that be-

126

cause our legs support and carry more weight, we develop stronger, more shapely leg muscles. The majority of the women I work with have very attractive legs—well shaped, strong, and with great muscle definition.

When I realized that my legs were a natural asset, I became vain about them and now take pride in keeping them in tip-top shape. I have extraordinary definition in my lower legs because they have been developed from the weight I carry and because I wear high heels a great deal.

High heels are a double-edged sword. They can help to tone and stretch the calf muscle but often are very bad for body alignment. As you are looking in the mirror, stand on your toes and look at the movement in your calf muscle. Do you see the muscles moving as you go up and down on your toes? Daily walking is what keeps your calves in shape more than anything else.

Do you dress to show off your legs or to conceal them? I often find that women who dislike their upper legs and thighs overcompensate and cover their entire leg—even if they have great lower legs and calves (lumping again!). Make a conscious effort to analyze which parts of your legs you do and do not choose to accentuate. Very, very rarely is there never a part of the well-rounded woman's leg to show off!

BODY PART 19: ANKLES

If you ask my friend Malissa what she believes the sexiest part of her body is, she will tell you her ankles. She also happens to have long legs, a great bustline, and a winning smile . . . but to her, the ankles win, no contest. I sometimes catch her looking down at her ankles—turning them from side to side, studying their shape and elegant bone structure. Even though she's far too modest and reserved to speak of her other assets, she'll always tell you how beautiful her ankles are. All I know about ankles I learned from Malissa.

Ankles can be shapely, sculptural, and elegant. Do as Malissa does and study your own ankles from every angle. When you are seated, look at the sides, the front, and the back as you rotate and circle them in the air. How do they look in panty hose? Smooth and defined? I know from having fractured my ankle last winter that there are hundreds of little bones that make up the ankle (much like the many little bones in our wrists.) The ankle is an intricate pivot point—strong and delicate at the same time. I don't recommend ankle bracelets—they break the continuous line of the leg and detract from the natural curves of the ankle and foot. Handle ankles with care. Once sprained or fractured, they are never quite the same again. Take it from Malissa, your ankles are worth the attention!

BODY POINT 20: FEET

Are you proud of your feet? Do you feel you can go barefoot without embarrassment? Do you give your feet the attention they deserve? Every women can have feet she is proud of. As we discussed in Step 3 (hands-on body rituals), our feet are overworked and underappreciated. Short of giving yourself the full home pedicure outlined in Step 3, hassle-free, well-maintained feet are achieved by following a few simple guidelines (a quick refresher course):

A pumice stone should be kept near the bathtub and be used on the bottoms and sides of the feet as well as the heels with *every* shower or bath. Toenails are kept short, clean, and clear of polish to avoid messy chipping.

Once a month (and as often as possible in the winter months) give yourself a deep-moisturizing treatment by generously lathering your feet with moisturizer and wearing cotton socks to sleep in, so the moisturizer sinks in. By adhering to these simple maintenance techniques, you can have attractive feet year-round.

Your feet absorb and transfer energy between your body and the earth. They are your connection to the ground—a physical point of entry and exit with the world in which you live. As your feet are carrying you through your world, check to see that you are moving *forward*, allowing your feet to guide you in a positive direction.

Use the Twenty-Point Body Map to remind you of your "positives" as you conduct your own assessment using the checklist found at the end of this step. And remember, you are much more than just a body. You are a perfect collection of all your inner and outer assets, capabilities, talents, and attributes. Work on the *inner* you first and the outer will naturally follow. As does the next step . . . where we will use our newfound assessment information to create a uniform.

1. Sharpen your assessment skills by observing other bodies. Notice how women "play up" their assets and downplay the rest.

2. Locate an accessible full-length mirror in your house. If you do not have one, please purchase one and install it in an unobstructed location where you can have privacy if you wish.

3. Using the Body-Positive Checklist, give yourself a head-to-toe assessment. In front of your full-length mirror, in your own private time, your own private space, and your own private way, assess each of your twenty body parts listed on the Body-Positive Checklist (add more as you discover them!). Remember, this does not have to be done overnight. Take as much time as you need, and refer back to the Twenty-Point Body Map descriptions as often as you wish.

4. List your newfound (or rediscovered) "positives." Complete this sentence, including the body parts you have listed in the "positives" column: "By taking the time to approach the mirror with acceptance and love, I have assessed my body and discovered that I like my _____ (list all your positives here!) _____ _____.

(Please continue listing on a separate sheet if needed!)"

MY BODY-POSITIVE CHECKLIST

	Accentuate	Downplay	Notes
Hair	_____	_____	_____
Eyes	_____	_____	_____
Lips/Mouth	_____	_____	_____
Nose	_____	_____	_____
Ears	_____	_____	_____
Neck	_____	_____	_____
Shoulders	_____	_____	_____
Arms	_____	_____	_____
Hands	_____	_____	_____
Back	_____	_____	_____
Chest	_____	_____	_____
Waist	_____	_____	_____
Lower Belly/Abs	_____	_____	_____
Hips	_____	_____	_____
Derriere	_____	_____	_____
Thighs	_____	_____	_____
Knees	_____	_____	_____
Lower Legs/Calves	_____	_____	_____
Ankles	_____	_____	_____
Feet	_____	_____	_____

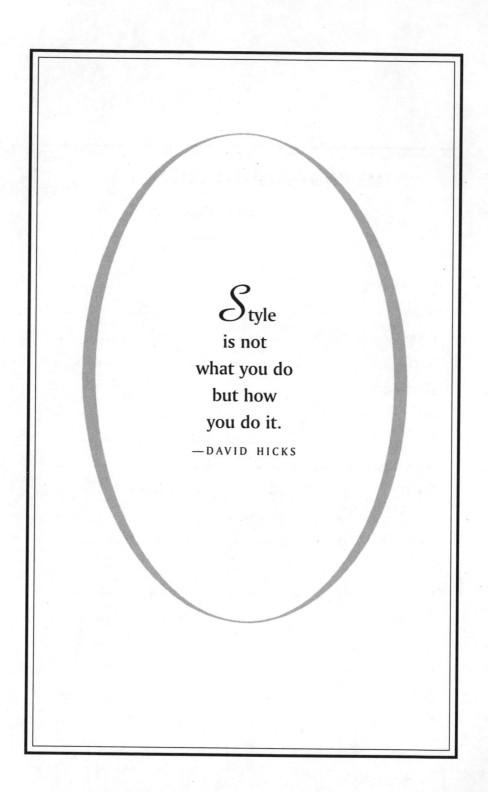

*S*tyle
is not
what you do
but how
you do it.

—DAVID HICKS

STEP

5

Create

a

Uniform

$\mathcal{W}$hat am I going to wear? Will it fit? What's clean? Will it be too tight? Too baggy? Did I forget to have it altered? Can I wear last year's short skirts this year? If it's not hot and it's not cold, what do I wear? Will I be able to breathe when I sit down? Am I wearing black too much? Will I be too hot if I keep my jacket on to cover my hips? Do I have to wear heels? Can I leave the top button undone? Does it make me look fat?

Why is getting dressed so hard? If it makes you feel any better, *you are not alone.* In fact, the above "gripe list" came from a *size 10* friend of mine when I asked her what her biggest fashion nightmares were. How interesting that so many of her answers are the exact same concerns I hear from women of size across the country and problems I have experienced firsthand myself! So there you have it . . . it's universal. We *all* worry about the same things when it comes to getting dressed.

Take my great friend Jane, for example. Jane and I are shopping buddies. I have learned a great deal from shopping with Jane. Jane is thirty-four years old, lives in Boston, and wears a size 4. Yes, you read it correctly, a size 4. The only time I had seen a size 4 on a label (before I met Jane) was on those circular racks in stores with the little plastic size dividers. The largest size (16 or 18) is always next to the smallest size (4 or 6). Occasionally when shopping for the 16s or 18s, a size 4 will be stuck in there by mistake. Twice a year, Jane and I take a trip together to the outlet mall. In the fall we trek northwards to Maine and in the spring we head for the Florida Panhandle.

From our many outlet experiences, I have learned that finding clothes is just as difficult for Jane as it is for us. I always thought that if you wore a size 4 or 6, you had it made in the shade . . . that the world was your own personal shopping mall. I thought you could walk in a store, put on anything, and it would look great. I was wrong. Jane, like every woman, needs a system and a plan for looking good. The rules for size 4 are the same as for size 24.

In this step, you will learn how to answer that one annoying question, "What do I wear?" The answer is actually quite simple and it is organized in a way that makes it easy for you to follow. You are about to begin operating on a new plane. A new level of dressing. A new personal system of style no matter what size you wear.

The "Big" Secret

Are you prepared to hear the big, huge secret shared among and guarded by the best-dressed women in the world, including fashion designers, fashion magazine editors, fashion industry professionals, and fashion models? This is the key that makes getting dressed and looking great easy. This is the secret that the entire fashion industry keeps to themselves.

This secret can be summed up in a single, Zen-like saying I once heard. Here it is: *"The more you know . . . the less you need."* Truly well-dressed women (and men) have pared down their wardrobe to the *essentials*—a *uniform*.

136

With their uniform, they have found the patterns, themes, and styles that work best for their bodies and their lifestyles, and they rarely deviate from it. It's all about finding a personal proven formula and *sticking to it.*

Now that you know the secret, you might be able to figure out why the fashion industry has shied away from sharing with us the key to effortless dressing. They enjoy the benefits of their own uniforms but hesitate to let the rest of us in on it, as they fear it will create an organized, educated, calm, confident customer. How can they sell the "latest" electric-blue-waif-vamp-pushed-up-corseted-grunged-sequined-long-skirt/short-skirt to a calm, focused customer who has a system and sticks to it? What they fear most is that our excessive, disorganized, fashion-victimized, panic purchases will cease. They're right. Once we learn to adhere to a well-thought-out system, there will be no more panic purchasing. We will begin purchasing with a vision and a plan.

But here's the flip side of the coin that I believe the fashion industry is missing. A customer who has created a uniform for herself is probably more interested in quality than quantity. She will wisely and happily spend *more* money to purchase something that is beautifully well made and will last for years.

The fashion industry does not have to suffer because of an educated consumer. In fact, in the long run, they will benefit by sustaining a *repeat* customer who comes back again and again to purchase her uniform "staples." Many smart designers know this, and as a result they create cohesive, relevant, well-constructed collections each season. Now you know the secret. You have the information. Keep reading to discover how to make this information work in your own life and your own closet!

What Is a "Uniform"?

Different people conjure up different images when they hear the word "uniform." I went to private school and wore a tartan plaid uniform every single day. I didn't realize how lucky I had it—not having to think about what I was going to wear for twelve years! Perhaps it was during this period, between the ages of six and eighteen, that the uniform system of dressing was ingrained in my way of thinking. The principle is the same. *A uniform is a constant:* finding out what works for you and repeating it; wearing variations of the same thing; discovering which clothes work well for your lifestyle and *confidently* duplicating that pattern over and over, adding subtle variations to keep things fresh from season to season.

Why We Need a New System for Dressing

My closet used to be a mess. I bought clothes randomly and haphazardly, choosing items just because they *fit* and not because I needed them. I had no game plan, no strategy, and no idea what to wear. I spent thousands of dollars on new clothes that hung in my closet with their tags still attached. I was known for making panic purchases—quickie, unplanned, random buys motivated by fear and deprivation. Fear of never being able to find something that would fit my body again, and the deprivation that comes from having only a limited (or nonexistent) selection of attractive, affordable clothes. The end result was that my closet was jammed with expensive, ill-fitting, mismatched clothes and I still had nothing to wear, and no system to rely on to put it all together. Sound familiar? I went through years existing in this state of fashion chaos.

Several years ago, I came to the conclusion that there *had* to be a better way. I decided to approach dressing myself in an orderly, strategic manner, utilizing my strengths and creating a system to simplify the process of getting dressed. I have based my system on the concept that *form follows function.* Form follows function simply means that what we wear (form) should be guided by what our lives demand (function). I am sharing my foolproof system with you, and by following this simple plan, you will reap the same benefits of one of my personalized one-on-one consultations. Follow along and free yourself from fashion purgatory!

In order to dress well every day and at any size, it is necessary to create a uniform . . . your own complete, calculated system for dressing based on your lifestyle needs, and covering all the bases from car pool to cotillion. Your personally tailored uniform system will bend, flex, grow, adapt, ease in, ease out, and move with your body and your lifestyle. It will be able to offer you viable, stylish options on any given day, including the days you feel tired, days you feel "puffy," days you feel sick, or days you just feel blah.

I am going to walk you through the process of uncovering your own uniform. You might have anywhere from one to five or six uniforms depending on your lifestyle. You may, for instance, have one for weekdays, one for weekends, and one for special events and parties. Of course, there are several versions of each of your uniforms for summer and winter climates.

The idea is to isolate and identify the types of clothing that accentuate your positives, make you look and feel great, and offer flexibility and consistency. Your uniforms will be the backbone of your wardrobe. Once they are established, you can add variety or season-to-season changes by utilizing accessories (see next step for more on accessorizing). When you have your uniform you will be able to dress with confidence, knowing what is right for your body and what will allow you to look your best!

How It Works

Discovering your uniform is easy. It involves a simple formula: $D^3 + C^3 = \text{Uniform}$.

Define your lifestyle patterns

Decode what those patterns mean in terms of the way you dress

Document emerging patterns in single words or phrases

Concentrate on your positives

Clear the clutter

Collect new items

Let's walk through each one and get your clothes organized once and for all!

DEFINE YOUR LIFESTYLE PATTERNS

Using the pages provided in the Toolbox at the end of this step, I want you to write down your clothing needs for three different but typical real-life scenarios. Make each scenario representative of how your life unfolds. Try to generalize what you do on a regular basis—whether it is going to work, taking care of your kids, going out to dinner regularly, or running errands. The idea here is to identify three (or more) of the most typical scenarios in your life. I will use myself (from a couple of years ago) as an example to show you what I mean.

Catherine's Scenario #1

Weekdays. Go to work. (I was an executive in a television public relations office.) I have to get dressed quickly in the mornings because I rush to the office after I do an early A.M. visit to the gym.

Catherine's Scenario #2

Weekends. Take a walk or a run in the mornings. Do errands. Shopping. I use Saturdays and Sundays to run around town, getting things done that I didn't have time to do during the week. I usually meet a friend for lunch on either or both days.

Catherine's Scenario #3

Dressy evenings out. Either weekday or weekend nights. Usually "cocktail party" dress required.

That's all there is to it. Just describe what it is you do on three different (but average) days. This information is the basis upon which we will begin to organize your personal uniform. I have provided the framework for you to make your own descriptive scenarios in the Toolbox following this step.

DECODE YOUR LIFESTYLE PATTERNS

Now that you have defined what it is that you typically do in three average situations, you are going to go one step further and use the space below to uncover or "decode" what *types* of clothing you typically choose to wear in each of those three situations. I want you to take a look at each of the three scenarios you just described, and decode what your lifestyle patterns mean in terms of how you dress. Follow along with my example.

Catherine's Decoding #1

Weekdays. For work on the weekdays I need to know what I am going to wear before I get dressed, because I'm always late and in a hurry. I want to be comfortable, but not sloppy. I wear black a great deal—it's flattering and doesn't show mistakes (ink, spots from lunch, city grime, etc.). I do not like to wear suits or fitted blazers—way too confining. I wear cotton blouses or shirts because if I wear silk or a silky fabric, I will always get a stain on it first thing in the morning! I like to wear slacks or skirts that I can move my legs in. I love days when I can wear my cashmere sweaters, or shawls—they make me feel secure and "cozy."

Catherine's Decoding #2

Weekends. I'm running around town and want mo-bility and comfort, without looking sloppy. I usually wear black leggings for most of the weekend. I exercise in the morning and sometimes have the urge to stay in my workout clothes all day because they are so comfortable. No hose, no skirts, no heels are the general rules for my weekends. But I have trouble with those rules when I have to meet someone for a nice lunch on Saturday when I need to look stylish but don't want to dress up.

Catherine's Decoding #3

For dressy occasions, I want comfort (yet again!) and ease of movement. I always wear black for cocktail and dressy affairs. It's chic, and always acceptable. Some-times I wish I could wear long dresses for the dramatic effect, but I never, ever have occasion to do so. No one wears long anymore. I use accessories to dress up otherwise simple outfits.

Get the picture? All you do is become more specific about the types of clothing you wear for your three typical scenarios. Give it a try by filling out your own decoding exercise in the Toolbox.

DOCUMENT THE EMERGING PATTERNS

We're almost there! You have defined and decoded. Now it's time to document the emerging patterns or trends that you have discovered in simple, one-word descriptions. I want you to zero in on the *key words* and *phrases* that you have used in your decoding. Lift these words out of the Decode boxes and write them down. In my decoding example, I have italicized words that I have lifted and used below. We are honing in very closely on your own personalized uniform and will use these descriptive words to categorize how you dress. Follow my example once again.

Catherine's Documentation #1

Quick. Comfortable. Black. Cotton. Pants. Skirts that I can move my legs in. Cashmere.

There! I've just zeroed in on one of my uniforms! These few words describe everything I need to know about how I want to dress for this scenario. Now all I have to do is fill in the blanks, describing my favorite pieces that fit this pattern.

Using these few words, I match them to *what already exists in my closet*—even if it is only *one* outfit, *one* skirt, or *one* blouse. These words are describing my short, pleated, *black skirt,* my *pants;* worn with one of my many *men's cotton dress shirts* (crisp and starched) or one of my *cashmere* sweaters. By spelling it out this way, I realize that this combo can work for every season. I wear the short, pleated skirts in wool for the winter and the same skirt in a linen/rayon blend for the warmer months. Same with the pants. Wool in the winter, linen in the summer, but always a dark color. I can layer one of my cashmere sweaters over the man-tailored shirt when it is cooler, or wear the cotton shirt alone when it warmer. Okay, let's look at my second scenario.

> ─────── *Catherine's Documentation #2* ───────
>
> *Mobility. Comfort. Casual. Black leggings. Stylish.*

To me this translates into *leggings* in a *dark color* (black or brown) paired with a *white T-shirt* and an easy *nonconstricting blazer* (I have a generously scaled navy blazer that covers my tummy and rear end) or leggings with an *oversized, A-line shirt* that also covers my tummy and rear end. I own one good white, oversized shirt that covers everything it is supposed to. When I keep the weekend uniform this simple, I can add a *big scarf* or *bigger earrings* to achieve a pulled-together, stylish look suitable for running errands and lunching with friends! And, finally:

> ─────── *Catherine's Documentation #3* ───────
>
> *Comfort. Ease of movement. Black. Long (?).*
> *Accessories.*

For evenings out, I want an easy yet elegant answer—a uniform from which I deviate very little. There's nothing worse than the feeling when you are invited out and need "special occasion" clothes and immediately fly into a panic about what to wear. I want to know that I am "covered" for any special event or evening that might arise, that there's a simple yet chic answer waiting for me in my closet!

For me, these few words and phrases helped me to recognize how much I love the comfort of my *chiffon pallazzo pants* (with stretch waist!). Very full and easy to wear, I own them in *black* and *white.* Instead of worrying over dress length, bugle beading, crystal pleating, or sequins, I create an *evening uniform* out of my basic chiffon pants. They are cut full in the leg and look like a *long skirt.* The way I achieve some variety is by keeping the pants the same and changing the top. I have one *lightly beaded top,* and several dressy long-sleeved *cashmere* and *cotton sweater tops.* On one of them I replaced the buttons with rhinestone and pearl ones to dress it up a little. Rows and rows of pearls are a staple in my evening uniform. I buy long strands of fake pearls and wear them either choker style or long and loose depending on the outfit. It *is* possible to have a special event/special evening uniform ready and waiting!

That's how simple it is. Now go back to your own decoding and look for the simple words and phrases that describe how you dress and write them in spaces provide in the Toolbox.

CONCENTRATE ON YOUR POSITIVES

At this point, you have successfully analyzed your lifestyle patterns, decoded them in terms of how you dress, and documented the emerging patterns in simple one-word or short-phrase descriptions. It is now time to pull in what we learned in the last step (Step 4: "Assess Your Outer Strengths"). I want you to bring to mind all the positives you rediscovered in the last step and apply them to the choices you make about your uniform.

Glance back at your Body-Positive Checklist and look through the "accentuate (+)" column. Go down the list and jot down the positives that you see. Wherever possible, use your positives to guide the choices you make while constructing your uniform. For example, if you have noted your lower legs and ankles as positives, be sure that within your uniform, you have chosen the proper skirt length to accentuate them. If it's your chest and neck you are proud of, make it a point to choose necklines that flatter and highlight your assets. If you love your eyes, choose to wear colors that showcase them close to your face. My uniform is mindful of my best asset—my legs. I wear shorter-length skirts and/or fitted leggings to show them off.

Celebrate your positives when you define your uniform. Accentuating your assets and downplaying the rest is the key to dressing well and feeling confident!

CLEAR THE CLUTTER

It means exactly what it says. Get rid of *all* the fashion mistakes, *all* the panic purchases, *all* the clothes that don't fit, *all* the miscellaneous pieces, and *all* the mismatched, random items gathering dust in your closet.

A uniform closet is a well-organized, tidy closet. It has a method, a purpose, a function, and a design. The only way to uncover your uniform is to get rid of everything that you know is *not* part of it. How do you know? Well, let me give you three simple guidelines for how to know what to get rid of things.

- *If you haven't worn it in a year . . . get rid of it.*
- *If you try it on and can't get it zipped, buttoned or fastened, get rid of it.*
- *If you are saving it for when you lose weight, get rid of it.*

147

If you adhere to these guidelines, your closet should emerge clutter free, with only uniform items left. Getting rid of it doesn't mean you have to throw it in the trash (unless it is ragged, tattered, torn, and generally unwearable.) Give your clothes to someone who can wear them right now, like a friend or a neighbor. My dressmaker wore the same size I did, so I would offer her my clothes, which she would either take for herself or pass along to someone else. Or you can donate them to a local church thrift store, sell them to a secondhand dress shop, or give them to Goodwill Industries or the Salvation Army. Many consignment shop owners I have spoken to are in need of more designer plus-size clothing in good condition. You will usually get back about half of the price it sells for in consignment.

Clearing the clutter from your closet will illuminate your real uniform. You must get rid of everything that is not currently functional in your closet. Now that you have discovered your uniform, clearing through the rubble of past fashion disasters will allow it the space to work and grow for you.

COLLECT NEW ITEMS

Collecting new items happens only after you have fully uncovered your uniform and cleared the clutter from your closet. This should *not* be confused with permission to go on a mad shopping spree. Collecting new items is the well-thought-out process of adding *essential* elements to your existing uniform.

Before you begin a quest for new uniform items, I encourage you to do some shopping in your own closet. Now that you have cleared the clutter, you can get a better look at what is left behind. What *should* be left is the foundation for one or more of your uniforms.

Take a second look at every item of clothing that has even the slightest chance of becoming part of your uniform. I call them "contenders." Pull out your contenders, and if they fit, take the time to give them a good, hard look. Sometimes all a jacket needs is new buttons, or a favorite skirt needs to be shortened a few inches. See how many of your existing clothes you can turn into part of your new uniform(s).

It's time to make a list. Two lists, actually. One is called your "More" list and the other is your "New" list. First, study the clothes you have and begin making a *detailed* list of the types of uniform essentials you would like to have *more* of—listing those items you discovered really worked for you, and ones whose concept or pattern you wish to repeat. For instance, your More list could sound like this: "more wide-leg pants with a stretch waist," or "more stretch leggings in dark colors," or "more cotton sweaters that cover my stomach and rear," or "more A-line dresses."

Now it's time to create your New list. This is an ongoing list that will change and grow as you discover "new" items that will work with your uniform. The "new" items are pieces that you have decided will work for you and your lifestyle, although they might be something you have never owned before. For instance, perhaps you discovered through the assessment process that you want to show off your upper back, and you realize that you have no clothes in your closet that accomplish that. This is something that would go onto your New list—"sweaters or tops that have a plunging or low back."

The New list, however, is where many of my clients get into a little trouble. They make the mistake of seeing something, immediately wanting it, and rushing to buy it, and *force* it to fit their uniform. The New list should be approached in the same orderly, thought-out manner as the More list. Care and planning to create a well-organized list will lead to a better, more efficient, and stylish uniform.

A few final thoughts on lists. Try to carry your list with you at all times. I keep a copy of my list folded up in my wallet, easily accessible wherever I go. You never know when you will find an opportunity to collect new items for your uniform. Having your list handy will eliminate random, thoughtless purchases.

When shopping to enhance your new uniform(s), I have found that it always pays in the long run to buy *quality* clothing. I would rather you buy just *one* beautifully made, quality skirt that works well in your uniform than three or four so-so ones. Well-made garments will last for years, stretching from season to season. The merits of how a quality garment *looks, feels, and lasts* outweigh cheap, quick purchases of clothing of lesser quality.

Money is a concern for all of us these days. There's no room to be wasteful or extravagant. Most women tell me that once they get their uniform system down pat, they save money. Uniforms can (and should) be constructed over time, not overnight. Don't throw everything away and try to start over immediately. Great uniforms grow slowly. Think things out. Add one beautiful piece at a time. Save up. Refuse to purchase anything if you are in a panic or frenzy. Uniform dressing should save you both time *and* money in the long run.

Size 2 or 22 . . . Who Cares?

Numbers and math have always given me trouble. I never related to numbers, numerical formulas, or algebraic equations. Sizes are just numbers. In fact, I find sizes *more* confusing than logarithms. As much as we live in a size-conscious world, sizes basically don't mean a thing. If anything, they are gross, approximate calculations based on ever-changing standards and guidelines.

References to "size," however, are omnipresent when we talk about clothes. "What *size* do you wear?" "What *size* are those pants?" "Do you have this in a bigger/smaller *size?*" "I got married in a *size* ten." "She's gone up three *sizes.*" "I'll try to squeeze into a smaller *size.*" Size is just a number on a dress label. Your size is probably different on many different pieces of your clothing. If it's not, it should be. Size is not a reflection of your self-worth, your self-esteem, your sense of humor, your intellectual capacity, or your capacity to love or be loved. Sizes are arbitrary numbers that shift and change with every garment you wear. Don't get caught up on a size. Sizes lie.

A recent article in *USA Today* reported that designers are "downsizing" more than ever. "Downsizing"? Let me explain. In an effort to entice sales, a designer will make a "size 12" dress and sell it with a label that says "size 10." Downsizing has become a popular practice because women like to think that they are buying (and wearing) a smaller size. "It's a feel good thing," states the article. Ridiculous but true. As a result, the science of sizing has gone down the tubes. Although it was never an exact science, there exists a set of standards and measurements which designers have used and accepted as guidelines for sizing throughout the years. But in light of downsizing, those standards have become obsolete. Who knows what size anyone is really wearing anymore? And in my opinion, who cares? Sizes don't matter—what looks good *does* matter.

I had an interesting experience modeling last spring.

I was working a trunk show in an upscale department store's plus-size department. I was modeling a single line of clothing over a three-hour period. The line was brand new and the department didn't have all the clothing in all the sizes in stock yet, and as a result I found that the eight outfits I was going to model ranged in size from a 14 to a 22. The amazing part of this story is that they all more or less fit. I'm not saying that some didn't fit better than others. They did. But I was able to wear a long, flowy skirt with an elastic waist in a size 14. In the trousers, I looked best wearing the size 18. And the size 22 belted jacket looked relaxed, easy, and comfortable.

The message here is that even within *one* line of clothing by the *same* designer, you can wear a multitude of different sizes. And it doesn't make a bit of difference which size you wear. Different garments fit different people differently. Find what looks and feels the best, and ignore the size label. If you feel compelled to glance at a size, go ahead and do so. But please look at it with an educated eye and smile to yourself, knowing you will ultimately choose to wear what looks and feels the best.

I recall a model I worked with many years ago. She more or less wore a size 16 and was completely caught up in the "size" game. Known in the market as sort of a "complainer," she *insisted* that she only be given size 16s to model, and if she were given anything larger, she took it as a personal affront. She had the idea in her head that being a 16 (whatever that means!) was "better" than being a size 18, 20, or larger. She would cause a commotion if she were given other sizes to wear, regardless if they looked better or not. I felt so sorry for her—pinning her self-worth on what size she wore.

My final advice is to try to use sizes as general, approximate guideposts, and nothing more. Release yourself from size purgatory, and concentrate on how clothing looks and feels on your body. I guarantee your wardrobe and your attitude will change for the better!

What's Your Signature?

Before I tell you what a "signature" is, let me ask you a few simple questions. If you had to describe how talk-show host Sally Jesse Raphael looks, what image immediately comes to mind? Her red glasses, right? How about Katharine Hepburn? Her trademark trousers and men's shirts combination. And former First Lady Nancy Reagan? Exactly. . . she was known for wearing red, red, red. And speaking of First Ladies, how about Barbara Bush? Her photograph has been taken hundreds of times with her signature triple-strand pearl necklace. How about Elizabeth Taylor? Aside from her infamous jewelry, she is recognized for her signature color—violet—matching her violet eyes. These are all personal trademarks or "signatures," as I like to call them—something uniquely special about the way a person dresses or looks.

Anything can potentially be a signature. It can be a signature color, a signature accessory, or a signature hairstyle. Signatures are important because they enhance your uniform(s), marking them with your own personal stamp or identity. You probably already have a signature without even knowing it—most of us do. The best way to discover your signature is to ask someone close to you this question: "When you conjure up an image of me, or how I dress, what do you think of?" You will be surprised to discover that the person you ask won't have much trouble coming up with something—whether it is the way you wear your hair, your "funky" shoes, or your colorful silk scarves.

For example, there is a very well-known French fashion designer who is known for her turtles. She collects "turtle" jewelry, mostly pins, which she wears daily. She is known for wearing her turtle pins on her clothes, but not just as the traditional shoulder pin. She will wear one perched on a sleeve at the wrist or even crawling up a hipbone on a pair of slacks! Her turtles are omnipresent and joyfully expected wherever she goes by everyone she knows!

I began wearing my two gold-link bracelets over five years ago. I never take them off because the clasps are difficult to open and close, so I just left them on day and night, night and day, in the shower, in the ocean, modeling, and traveling. As a result, five years later, I feel positively naked without my matching gold-link bracelets. They are a part of me and all my uniforms. It sort of happened by accident, but now I have chosen to keep them as a Catherine Lippincott signature.

You may find you have one signature or perhaps several. Your signature is uniquely yours and is a method of owning your uniform, creating your own look and individual style.

More Tips, Hints, and Secrets of Seventh Avenue

I want to share with you *everything* I know about how to dress well in any size. Many of these ideas have come from my work in the fashion industry—on the runways, in the showrooms, and working with the designers. Read them, use them, share them with friends, and be sure to write me and let me know *your* tips, hints, and secrets that I can share with other well-rounded women!

ALTERATIONS ARE THE RULE, NOT THE EXCEPTION

I have learned to be a master of "fix it, hem it, cut it off, let it out, take it in." The very plain fact of the matter is that alterations are the *rule*, not the exception, for *all women*.

Think about it in these terms. The purest form of dressing the body (and the most expensive) is haute couture. Haute couture involves custom cutting and sewing clothes to fit a body. Haute couture is practiced in France, where a very small percentage of the female population travels to have their clothes made to the exact shape and size of their bodies. A daytime suit or dress can (and in most cases *does*) cost as much as $20,000. Yes, that's twenty thousand dollars. In actuality there are only a handful of women *in the world* who pay for couture. Everything else that *everyone* else wears is considered ready-to-wear.

Ready-to-wear is premade, mass-manufactured clothing designed in the most universal way possible to fit as many bodies as possible. And as we know, no two bodies are alike, no matter what their size. When you look at it this way, it's only logical that all our clothes should require alterations.

Men understand this concept better than women. They have been very well trained to *expect* alterations. And you had better believe that they don't blame themselves or their bodies when something doesn't fit right off the bat. A man just bellows for "alterations" to come running and fix it. In fact, the idea of walking out of a

155

store with a new suit under his arm is not even part of his reality. Men are generally followed *into the dressing room* by the alterations person, who takes measurements and pins and tucks to create a perfect fit. Women can learn from men in this area. Alterations don't mean you are abnormal or have an unusual body. They are to be expected if you expect a good fit.

TRY TO RECYCLE OR "FIX" WHAT YOU ALREADY HAVE

Many times we have clothes in our closet that need some fixing. Often I change the buttons on an older blazer to add a little new pizzazz. Other times all a skirt needs is to be shortened or tapered to the knee. I have been known to take an old dress with a round neckline (unflattering on me) and have it made into a V-neck. As a result, I have a seemingly "new" dress that I *will* wear now that it is more suited to my body and what looks flattering on me.

As you are clearing the clutter from your closet, take a good, hard look at each article of clothing. Picture it in your mind with a slight change or alteration. Ask yourself if there is anything that you could do to that shirt, skirt, or dress that would make it new and exciting and an element that would fit nicely into one of your uniforms.

CHOOSE A SIMPLE SHAPE OR PATTERN THAT WORKS FOR YOU AND KNOCK IT OFF "LINE FOR LINE"

If you have an article of clothing that you love, knock it off! By this I mean take it to an experienced dressmaker and have it used as a pattern for other garments. For instance, if you just adore the simple red dress you wore to a wedding last year, take it to your dressmaker with an armful of new fabrics and have her make the same dress over and over, line for line, in a dozen different fabrics, colors, and patterns.

If you love the way something looks, fits, and feels, *please, please, please* make the investment of having it replicated, so you can wear your favorite dress (or a version of it) every day. A sure thing is a sure thing!

CREATE A LONG-TERM WORKING RELATIONSHIP WITH A TAILOR OR DRESSMAKER

Speaking of dressmakers, this point naturally follows the last. However, if you *yourself* are a master of the needle, you can skip this tip altogether. This tip is for any of us who are unable to sew on a button.

As discussed above, alterations are the rule, not the exception. It only makes sense for all well-dressed women to have in their back pocket someone who knows their body and can take care of all their alterations and dressmaking needs. Once you have found someone whose work you like and whom you trust, you have conquered half the battle! Your altering needs might range from shortening a skirt or dress to reshaping the lines of a jacket. Make sure your seamstress can also handle your needs for having clothes made from the patterns you find and like.

Once you have established a relationship and have together created two or three patterns of simple, great shapes, all you will have to do is pick out the fabric you want something made in, and drop it off! What could be easier? I even leave my patterns with my dressmaker, so I don't have to dig them out every time I need something new made.

Well Rounded

LEARN THE IMPORTANCE OF A FEW GOOD NEUTRALS

If versatility and flexibility are important to you, build your uniforms around a few good neutral-colored garments. By *neutral* I mean blacks, browns, navy blues, grays, and tans. If you stick to the neutral color palette, you will get more for your money—neutrals are *much* more versatile than other colors. You can mix neutrals with many other colors or add a much trendier accompanying piece to a neutral one and get a totally different look.

With neutrals, less *always* looks like more. You can get many more combinations out of a single neutral-colored suit as compared to, say, a floral patterned one. Neutrals also lend an air of elegance and restraint. Well-made, classic, neutral pieces last a lifetime.

HAVE A STACK OF CLEAN, PRESSED WHITE T-SHIRTS

As simple as it sounds, a white T-shirt is a uniform staple. Pressed white T-shirts look terrific with suits, skirts, or trousers for a pared-down, classic look. A simple white T-shirt can be just the touch you are searching for to go with many different uniforms or looks. When a white T-shirt is worn under a classic neutral-colored suit instead of a silk blouse it lends a modern edge to the whole look.

Your white T-shirts must be void of any color, design, or logo and preferably of a good heavy cotton stock (so you don't have to worry about see-through problems.) I iron my T-shirts to give an ever crisper look. Buy your T-shirts large enough so that they do not cling to your body at any point.

An added bonus of white T-shirts is that they feel so great next to your skin. Cotton helps to keep you cool! In addition, white is great when worn close to the face, because it acts a backdrop for your smile and your expressions. The idea here is to look pared down, clean, modern, and comfortable.

INSIST ON GOOD FOUNDATION GARMENTS

As you probably already know, this is not as easy as it sounds. Underwear and foundation garments are still difficult to find in plus sizes. But a little persistence and determination will pay off in ways that might surprise you. I have discovered that women who do not have the proper bras, panties, slips, all-in-ones, and so on are compromising how great they can look. Good foundation allows our clothes to fit better and *look* better as a result.

More so than our smaller-sized sisters, women of size need quality foundation garments. Simply stated, we have more to lift and support. Fit is essential in purchasing your foundation. In order to ensure a correct fit, you may want to have a fitting or consultation with an expert. Locate the store (or stores) in your area that carry foundation garments in larger sizes. I am pleased to report that many department stores around the country are carrying a better selection of larger sizes than ever before.

Ask questions and make sure your consultation is with an experienced professional who knows the exact science of fitting women for foundation garments. She will more than likely come into the dressing room with you, take measurements, ask you some preliminary questions, and bring back some items for you to try. Occasionally, women tell me that they find this process "embarrassing," and they hesitate to go through with it. I can assure you that it is worth a little lack of modesty to ensure that you are wearing the proper foundation.

Since we are speaking frankly, I'll share my personal

choice of undergarments with you. I have been wearing all-in-one foundation garments for almost fifteen years. All-in-ones (like a supportive "body suit") are available in a multitude of sizes, shapes, styles, and price ranges. I feel I am most comfortable in an all-in-one because it gives me support while creating a smooth, clean line underneath my clothes. I most often wear a beautiful lacy one that has the all-essential underwire and comes up to a size 40DD (see the Resources section at the end of the book). I wear all-in-ones with everything and for every occasion. I have one for active wear, one for sheer clothes, and even a strapless one for a shoulder-baring evening outfit I own.

Some women I work with don't like all-in-ones and choose to wear a well-fitted bra. Again, I am happy to report that the top manufacturers of foundation and underwear garments are now providing a selection of attractive, well-made bras in plus sizes.

Whatever you choose as your foundation, make sure it is doing its job well. Your undergarments should be providing you with a smooth, supportive, and comfortable foundation for your clothes to cover. As an important health-related side note, properly fitted, quality foundation can assist in improving your posture and potentially alleviating back problems.

THERE IS A SOLUTION FOR THE MOST COMMON DISCOMFORT AMONG WOMEN OF SIZE

Very frankly, and without mincing words . . . our legs rub together. There. I said it. Living inside our bountiful bodies, we experience a thigh-friction problem. By wearing leggings or trousers in the winter months we can somewhat escape the trauma. (And if you have ever experienced the condition, "trauma" *is* the word for it. I wouldn't wish thigh rub on my worst enemy.) Let me offer a potential solution that I have found helpful.

The way to stop thigh rub is to alleviate friction between the legs. Powder works as a short-term solution. But for more lasting results, there is a better answer. Wearing cotton "legging shorts" underneath your clothing alleviates the rubbing—keeping your legs cool, dry, and comfortable. By "legging shorts" I mean the solid-color cotton leggings that stop just *above* your knee. They are sometimes referred to as "bike messenger pants," as every messenger in NYC wears a version of these above-the-knee leggings. (See Resources.)

The key here is to buy all cotton with only a touch of Lycra, as the shiny 100 percent Lycra ones tend to hold more heat. The cotton breathes. You can wear these under your skirts, baggy shorts, and over panty hose. Because they are so fitted to the leg, they create almost no visible lines underneath your clothing. They keep your upper thighs separated, dry, and frictionless. It works.

KEEP COMPLETE OUTFITS TOGETHER
FOR EASE OF DRESSING

I learned this trick from modeling. At a photo shoot or a runway show, the outfits to be modeled are neatly arranged, with each change pulled together on the hanger. This is done for ease, organization, and to help the model make her changes quickly, without forgetting anything, in spite of the sometimes frenzied rush of a show or shoot. Hanging with each outfit is the proper hosiery as well as all jewelry, scarves, handbag, and so on.

I learned how easy it was to get dressed effortlessly when all the "pieces of the puzzle" are hanging there together, and I now employ this technique in my own closet with the help of Margie's Bags. A Margie Bag (named for the woman who invented it) is a clear plastic wardrobe accessory bag that hangs with an individual outfit.

With three pockets of different sizes, the bag is a perfect place to keep your coordinating accessories together—everything from jewelry, scarves, and hair accessories to hats, caps, gloves, belts, hosiery, or small purses. Each bag has a steel-grommetted hole (to avoid tearing) at the top, which fits over the neck of a coat hanger. I accessorize an outfit on the hanger, so that I don't forget to wear those special earrings I bought to go with a certain dress, or so that I remember that my big black-and-white silk scarf looks great when used as a belt with my black wool trousers.

By keeping all the pieces together, I can get dressed in my favorite uniform with all the special touches without having to think! You can order Margie Bags for your own closet. (See Resources.)

BE A CREATIVE SHOPPER

Great clothing finds don't stop at the plus-size department. Women of size have had to be much more clever in sleuthing out clothes that fit and look good too, and we have learned to shop *everywhere* to find what we need. Necessity breeds invention, and here are some of my best-kept and inventive secret shopping destinations!

I bend the gender barriers by shopping at men's stores—both regular-size men's stores and departments as well as the big and tall men's shops. Men's stores offer several wardrobe items that work in my uniform as a well-rounded woman.

First, I look for oversized sweaters in wool, cotton, and cashmere. Men's sweaters are more generously cut than women's and often I buy them in XXL-Tall to get extra length to cover my stomach and rear. My second stop in the men's store is the shirt department, where I purchase beautiful pima cotton men's dress shirts, which I wear over leggings (nice long shirttails also cover the rear!). I sometimes purchase the shirts with French cuffs and wear stunning cufflinks for extra impact! Don't be shy about shopping in a men's store. Ask questions, try things on, and request a fitting room away from the others to ensure your privacy.

I love shopping in maternity stores. It took me years to become bold enough to go into one and now I chuckle each time the saleslady asks me, "When are you due, honey?" I never feel insulted because she asks *everyone* that same question—after all, it *is* a maternity shop! I just smile sweetly and knowingly and say, "Oh, I'm not pregnant. I'm just a very clever size sixteen shopper!"

Once I have established my reasons for being there, I scout for good finds. Although many of the maternity pants and skirts don't work (because of the special "belly panel" in front), I have found several good dresses in these specialty shops. In these modern days of the "working mom," maternity stores are carrying plenty of work dresses—which are usually dresses cut fuller through the midsection (without panels), including simple A-line shapes that float away from the belly area. In the past two years I have found several wonderful dresses at maternity shops, including a black, A-line party dress with marabou feather trim!

Women of size can find wonderful things in maternity shops. Sizewise, most of the shops I've been in carry items in S, M, L or XL. I find that the XL can fit up to size 20. Go take a look and see what you find!

I am a great proponent of outlet shopping. I find amazing bargains at the outlets and am increasingly encouraged by the number of plus-size retailers who are represented at the outlet malls. As I mentioned earlier, my friend Jane and I make a pilgrimage to the outlets twice a year. Do a little research and find out where the closest outlets are. Please be armed with an extra good list when you outlet shop. The endless rows of stores and incredible bargains can overwhelm and sidetrack even the most organized shopper.

CLOTHES SHOULD BE THE "STAGE" FOR YOUR PERSONALITY

A final tip of *paramount* importance. This is my way of describing the old adage, "Wear your clothes, don't let them wear you." Clothing should be kept to a well-fitted, stylish and appropriate minimum. You want to receive compliments like these: "You look beautiful tonight" or "You look fabulous!" rather than "Wow . . . what a dress." Your clothes should provide a beautiful backdrop to showcase your personality, your humor, your wit, your joy of life.

Fashion Faux Pas

As you are analyzing your uniform and your uniform needs, run through this final checklist to make sure you are not violating any of the fashion faux pas most common among well-rounded women.

FAUX PAS #1:
HAVING TOO MANY THINGS GOING ON AT ONCE

Unfortunately, many of the clothes available for women of size are complexly decorated with too many rhinestones, too much beading, fancy appliqués, lace borders, and intricate, elaborate buttons, trim, tassels, bows, and fringe. Instead of giving us clean, simple versatile pieces, designers of plus-size clothing oftentimes overdo the froufrous. Don't be shy about removing studs, dangles, or embroidery from the clothes you buy. You will look better for it.

Several years ago I bought a very expensive, well-made dress that was beautiful in every way except . . . the designer had big flower appliqués attached at the hem. As soon as I got it home, I carefully removed the appliqués and as a result, the dress is perfect! When you are shopping try to look *beyond* too many buttons or bows and decide if the garment would be better without them. Make sure you can successfully remove the excessive decoration without harming the garment.

Be mindful of keeping accessories to a clean minimum if you are wearing an elaborately designed suit, blouse, or dress. A good rule of thumb is to get completely dressed and then go back to the mirror and take one thing off. Women of size look best in simple chic instead of gaudy glitz.

FAUX PAS #2:
CLOTHES THAT ARE TOO TIGHT

Just don't do it. Tight clothes are a sign of cheap clothes. Kings and queens wore loose robes and flowy capes because it was the ultimate luxury to be able to afford all that fabric. Dress like a queen. There is no need to scrimp on size. Nowadays we can all afford to buy a size that fits and flows rather than constricts and binds.

Notice the subtle yet important difference between clothes that are "fitted" and clothes that are "tight." Fitted clothing can look good on women of all sizes. Tight clothing looks good on *no one*. Fitted clothing follows the line of the body without constricting movement, pulling, or tugging. Tight clothes are clothes that are simply the wrong size. This concept applies to knits and clingy fabrics as well.

Knits can look divine on a larger, more voluptuous woman provided she buys the correct size. I see many women who try to fit into a garment that they have long outgrown. By trying to squeeze into something, she is announcing to the world that she is in a state of denial about her body. Remember, we now know that sizes don't mean a thing. So buy what fits. If it's tight, take it off.

FAUX PAS #3:
CLOTHES THAT ARE TOO BIG

On the other hand, unless we are careful, clothes that are too big for us can make us look bigger than we actually are. Clothing should *fit*, without constricting, pulling, or binding *and* without hanging, drooping, or sagging. When women of size are wearing something far too big, they think they are hiding underneath the clothing. It doesn't work that way. If it's too big, it only makes you look bigger.

Otherwise attractive jackets look ill proportioned and messy if they are too large; a dress turns into an amorphous sack if it's too big for you, and oversized sweatshirts and T-shirts, in my opinion, only make you look oversized. Strive for clothes that allow ease of movement and a comfortable fit, but be cautious not to cross the line—trying to "hide" underneath clothing that is too large. This leads nicely into my next point . . .

FAUX PAS #4:
MISTAKING SLOPPY FOR "CASUAL"

I often find in my work that women tend to confuse "casual" with "sloppy." There are often occasions when casual attire is called for and should be a part of your uniform system of dressing. However, there is no occasion or situation that I can think of outside of the privacy of your house where sloppy dressing is appropriate. Old, baggy sweatpants with a T-shirt or sweatshirt is sloppy. A cotton sweater with matching pants is "casual." Today well-rounded women enjoy a more extensive selection of clothes, and with a little more effort and thought, we can successfully dress to look casual and comfortable without looking sloppy or unkempt.

FAUX PAS #5:
CREATING A "LINE" IN THE WRONG SPOT

The point at which an article of clothing "stops" on your body is exactly where the eye will be naturally drawn. Any horizontal line such as a skirt hem or the bottom of a jacket will attract attention to that area. I see many women who cannot figure out why an outfit makes them look larger than they are. It is usually because of where the horizontal line hits their body.

If you want to detract attention from your hips, wear jackets and tops that fall above or below your hip line.

It's the same for skirts. If you wish to detract attention from your lower legs and calves, wear skirts that hit either above or below the calf. Take note of what you want to accentuate and downplay and make sure the line crossing your body is at the most flattering point possible.

FAUX PAS #6:
UNFLATTERING NECKLINES

Generally speaking, women of size look better in necklines that elongate the body or frame the face such as a V neck or a "sweetheart" neckline. Even a turtleneck in a dark, neutral shade can frame the face dramatically. Where we run into trouble is with a traditional "jewel" or round neckline. Because a round neck stops just below the neck and just above the collarbone, it literally "chops off" our head. Necklines that fall above or below that plane tend to do better, elongating the body, framing the face, and creating a more attractive overall look.

FAUX PAS #7:
POCKETS OVER YOUR CHEST

I don't know why, but designers continue to make blouses, tops, and dresses that have pockets (sometimes even with a flap) over the chest. I have yet to see any woman of size on whom this is attractive. One big pocket over each side of our bosom only makes us look topheavy and pigeon-breasted! And there is no function for pockets over the chest for a woman. A man might have some reason to keep items in a chest pocket, but women do not.

If I want to purchase a blouse but it has pockets over the chest, I look carefully to see if there's any way they could be removed without damaging the garment. If not, I will generally *not* buy it.

It will take a little time and concerted effort to make uniform dressing part of your life but once you do, you will discover how easy getting dressed and looking great can be. Well-rounded women deserve to dress beautifully and hassle free. And, to embellish our uniform, we now move on to proper accessorizing.

T O O L B O X

5

1. Define your lifestyle patterns (see p. 140):

My Real-Life Scenario #1:

My Real-Life Scenario #2:

My Real-Life Scenario #3:

2. Decode what those patterns mean in terms of how you dress (see p. 142):

My Decoding #1:

My Decoding #2:

My Decoding #3:

3. Document the emerging patterns (see p. 143):

My Documentation #1:

In this real-life scenario, what can you glean from these simple words that relate to the clothes you have?_____
_____.

My Documentation #2:

In this real-life scenario, what can you glean from these simple words that relate to the clothes you have?_____
_____.

My Documentation #3:

In this real-life scenario, what can you glean from these simple words that relate to the clothes you have?_____
_____.

4. Go to your closet and clear the clutter. Remember the guidelines:

If you haven't worn it in a year . . . get rid of it.

If you try it on and can't get it zipped, buttoned, or fastened . . . get rid of it.

If you are saving it for when you lose weight . . . get rid of it.

5. Based on your findings in your closet, begin to make your lists for collecting items for your uniform.

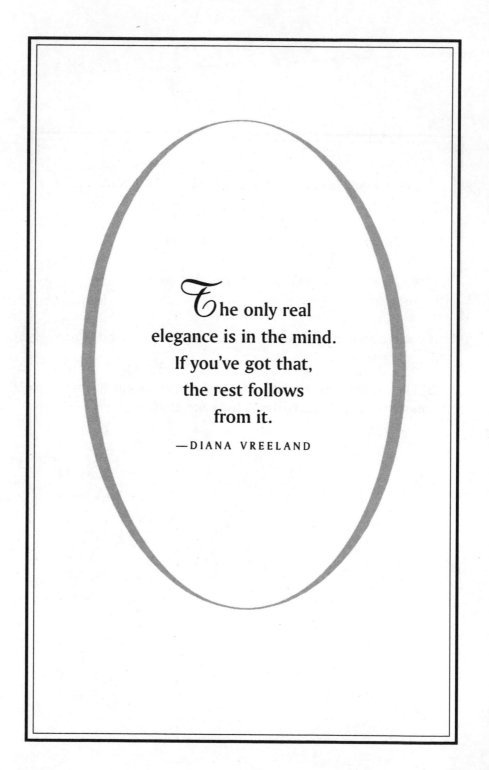

$\mathcal{T}$he only real
elegance is in the mind.
If you've got that,
the rest follows
from it.

—DIANA VREELAND

STEP

6

Accessorize Your Life Appropriately

*A*ccessories are the all-important details that either enhance or detract from the way we look. In this step I will show you how to choose the appropriate accessories to complement your well-rounded body. You will learn about "fashion" accessories such as jewelry, hats, scarves, and belts, and also what I call "life" accessories—anything that touches your life or has contact with your physical self, such as furniture, cars, "space," and more.

Before we get into actual baubles and beads, we must first address the larger issue—scale and proportion. Correct accessorizing demands attention to *proportion.* By definition, if something is *in proportion,* it is in a "proper or pleasing relation to another." Proportion is one of the most important principles in any of the arts, including the art of accessorizing.

Principles of Proportion

Imagine one of the great cathedrals in Europe if the architects or builders didn't mind the rules of scale and proportion. Buildings have a flow and harmony that is based on adhering to correct proportions. How about a classic painting or portrait? In order for a work of art to be pleasing to the eye, the artist uses the correct proportions and the balance of the composition to arrange elements on the space of the canvas. The same principle applies in your own living room. If you add a piece of furniture that is too large or too small for the size of the room, it completely throws off the continuity and flow of the space. Attention to proportion and balance is essential no matter what the object in question—a cathedral, a portrait, an interior, a dress, or your body.

A larger body does not necessarily mean every accessory we choose, fashion or otherwise, needs to be scaled up or possess larger-than-life proportions. In fact, as a general rule, accessories look best on women of size when they are proportioned somewhere between the teeny-tiny and the gargantuan. Tiny, dainty accessories get lost on our ample curves and the big, clunky ones can overpower us. On most of the women I work with, the medium-size range looks best. Correct proportions in accessorizing (as in everything we do!) help to organize elements in space or on our bodies, in an eye-pleasing manner.

Diva or Dud: How We Choose to Use Our Space

We all occupy space—some of us more, some less. As well-rounded women, I believe that we are privileged to have more space than our size 6 friends. The luxury of occupying more space is that we automatically make a statement every time we walk down the street or into a room. We don't have to say a word. Our bodies create an instant impact, have built-in drama, and demand attention. The next time you are at a party or gathering, notice how the more well-rounded woman turns heads when she enters the room, and how our smaller sisters enter virtually unnoticed.

I know what you're thinking. You are saying to yourself that the attention we attract when we enter a room might *not* be positive—that people are staring at us, and maybe not in a good way. Well, here's the responsibility part of the deal. For better or worse, people *are* looking. It's *our* responsibility to use that attention positively. This is the essence of the "diva or dud decision."

The "dud" chooses to schlump into a room, shuffling her feet, dressed in drab, unattractive clothing with her eyes cast down to the floor. The "diva," on the other hand, enters looking well groomed (if not drop-dead gorgeous!), standing up tall, confident, smiling and laughing, with an open attitude to new situations and new people—using every inch of her space to the fullest.

We have the responsibility of making the space we occupy the most pleasing, attractive, healthy, and vibrant we possibly can. We are responsible for keeping up, maintaining, celebrating, and adorning our space. Learning to accessorize our body properly is part of that adornment process.

Fashion Accessories

Fashion accessories are those elements we choose to enhance and complement our overall look. In this section, I will touch on six fashion accessory categories: jewelry, scarves, belts, hats and gloves, shoes, and handbags and purses. There exist, however, a few general guidelines that apply to *all* fashion accessories.

Test, try, and play. Test out a new way of wearing a scarf. Try belting a blouse. Play with several chains instead of just one. You have to experiment with fashion accessories to learn what is right for you. Look at the magazines. Pick up trends. Try them out on yourself. See what works. Use the mirror. Learn to trust your own eye. Does it feel right? Is the scale correct? Are you comfortable wearing it? These are the types of questions you should be asking yourself as you test out fashion accessories.

Accessorizing is not an exact science. Fashion "stylists," whose job it is to dress and accessorize models on photo shoots, are the best example. They will put a pair of earrings on a model, stand back and look, and then may whisk them off her. They scream, "Hold it! Don't shoot!" and run onto the set to retie a scarf or add another bracelet. They are the masters of "try it . . . and if it doesn't work, fix it or get rid of it!"

Scan the fashion magazines, tear out pages with looks that are attractive to you, and reproduce them in your own way. Remember, when you are testing, trying, and playing with accessories, always, *always* use a full-length mirror. You cannot get the full picture of what an accessory looks like on your body unless you can see it in relation to your whole body.

Find your accessory trademark and stick to it. This goes back in part to a concept we discussed in the last step. Find a signature accessory statement and stick to it. Nowhere in your wardrobe is it easier to create a signature look than with your accessories. Find an accessory (gold hoop earrings) or type of accessory (colorful oblong silk scarves) and adopt it as your own. See what you already have, and what you already enjoy wearing. Your trademark accessory should fit comfortably into your lifestyle, your uniform, and your look.

Jewelry

Wearing jewelry is a delightful and dramatic way to accessorize your look. Often women of size misuse the jewelry they have, because they believe it is only incidental to their look. In fact, it is just the opposite. Jewelry can draw wanted attention to precise body areas, as well as drawing it away from others. Women of size should know how to use jewelry properly to enhance their assets and create impact. I will break down jewelry into separate categories, but first, here are the two general jewelry rules for women of size that apply to all your jewelry!

JEWELRY RULE #1:
IT DOESN'T HAVE TO BE REAL

If you are one of the very few lucky women who own big, important, dazzling jewels, yippee! Wear them, showcase them, and by *all* means don't keep them forever hidden away in a safe. The point of having beautiful *real* stones is to wear them so that they can catch light and sparkle. That is their sole mission in life. Unless you are wearing them, they are not living up to the investment you made in them. However, if you are like the rest of us, and the only "rocks" you have are in your yard, read on!

Jewelry does not have to be real. Many of the women I work with are not utilizing jewelry as the wonderful fashion accessories they can be because they believe that jewelry has to be "real." Wrong. There is no law stating that we have to wear all *real* gold or *real* silver, *real* diamonds or *real* anything, and we should be glad, because most of the *real* we could honestly afford would be small and insignificant, lacking impact. These days, no one can tell the difference and no one cares. What looks good is what's right. There is a wide selection of gorgeous costume jewelry to choose from, available in every style and design you could wish for.

Jewelry, both real and faux, should have impact. And

to achieve that impact, the best solution is to mix the real with the faux. Mix it all up, make them wonder, keep them guessing, and never tell! Coco Chanel revolutionized this concept by designing faux jewelry that mimicked her real jewelry—and then wore them together!

We all have a few pieces of real jewelry. Perhaps it is your diamond engagement ring, a gold charm bracelet that belonged to your mother, or a pair of diamond stud earrings. Use these elements to mix with faux pieces. But try to get rid of any smallish, real jewelry that you don't wear or don't care about. Go through your real jewelry and select the pieces that have the most impact. Keep any jewelry that you can't bear to get rid of for sentimental reasons and sell the rest. I knew a lady who got tired of all her smallish real jewelry. She took each item, had all the stones removed (small diamonds, minuscule rubies, emerald bits, and sapphire chips), and designed one big dome ring with all the stones in it. She called it her "constellation ring" because all the little stones put together looked like stars and planets in the sky.

JEWELRY RULE #2:
BIG AND SIMPLE IS PREFERABLE TO SMALL AND INTRICATE

This rule goes hand in hand with the first. Generally speaking, if you stick to real jewelry it will lack *size and simplicity*—two of the most important concepts to remember in accessorizing well. A few well-chosen pieces of simple, nicely proportioned jewelry is all you need. Put on a pair of earrings, a pin, or a bracelet and then stand way back from a full-length mirror (at least twenty paces). Can you see the jewelry now? If you can see at least a glimmer or a shine from that far away, chances are you have chosen well and it has substantial proportions and sufficient scale so it will not get lost on your body, and lose its impact. Your jewelry should be the punctuation marks enlivening your uniform.

Too many women (of all sizes) err on the side of "small, sentimental, dainty" jewelry. Thin little chains dangling a tiny diamond chip only make our necks look bigger in comparison. Multiple rings with lots of small stones get lost on your hands. Earrings in the "shape" of things can be distinguished only on close inspection, not from a distance.

Nowhere is the importance of jewelry size and simplicity more apparent than in runway modeling. In order for jewelry to be seen on a model on a runway, it has to have impact and scale. A few bold strokes with sufficient size (one *big* pin) or the repetition of an element (ten stacked matching dangle bracelets instead of one or two) are devices used to create jewelry impact on the runway. Our daily life is not unlike life on the runway. We dress, we move, we strut, we want to make an impression. Remember: size and simplicity for each of the five jewelry categories: earrings, necklaces, pins, bracelets, and rings.

Earrings are the most important accessory for drawing attention to the face. Regardless which part of your face you want to highlight—your eyes, your rosy cheeks, a regal nose, or your smile—the right earrings can illuminate the feature of your choice! Earrings are arrows that point to your face, directing the eye to your facial expressions and movements. Earrings say, "Look right here, I want you to pay attention to what I am saying or expressing." Any woman's looks can be enhanced by the correct size and shape earring.

How do you find earrings that are right for you? Earrings should not be too small or too big. Try on all your earrings and see which ones look and feel the most natural. As discussed earlier, small earrings have the tendency to get "lost" on the body, and huge earrings can look awkward and clunky. I find that well-proportioned earrings in what would be considered the "medium" range look the best on most women of size.

All you need are the four basic earring types—the simple ball or button in gold or silver; a pearl *and* gold Chanelesque button or oval style; small hoops; and rhinestone "drops" or cubic zirconium solitaires for evening. (Cubic Zirconium solitaires can be for daytime too. A little sparkle or glimmer always lights up the face day or night. Make sure they are at *least* the equivalent of one carat in size to maximize sparkle!)

Of course you can add to these four basic earring styles, having variations on each type. Go to your jewelry box and divide your earrings into style groups. Try on each pair and check their condition. Nothing is more frustrating than reaching for a pair of earrings and discovering that a back is missing from a favorite pair of pierced earrings, or having a clip-on earring fall off because of a loose spring. Get rid of the broken, unfixable earrings taking up precious space, or take them to be repaired. Give away the earrings that you never wear and keep paring down until you left with only the earrings that you adore and are wearable!

A quick side note about earring shapes. You need to try all different shapes to find out what looks best on you, but here's something I've discovered from working with women of size. Depending on the shape of your face, we generally look better in *elongated* shapes. Instead of a perfect round circle, try an elongated circle, an oval. This applies to all earring styles, from "button" earrings to hoops. Round shapes reinforce other round shapes. Elongated shapes reinforce the *elongation* of the body.

Also take into consideration how you wear your hair when you are choosing the appropriate earring. You don't want long hair worn down to get caught in dangle earrings. With a short haircut that covers most of the ear, you might want something that *does* hang below the line of the hair so it can be seen.

I own just a few pair of earrings from each of the basic groups and make them work with each uniform. However, some women I work with just love to purchase earrings to complement a specific look or outfit. If you are among these women, be sure to make use of your clear plastic accessory bags and keep the earrings *with* the outfit they were purchased for. Why bother having so many "specialized" earrings if you are going to forget to wear them?

A necklace, like a pair of earrings, should bring the beholder's eye upward and illuminate the wearer's face. However, necklaces are a little more difficult to wear well. In more cases than not, women are wearing necklaces when they should not. In fact, when I work one on one with women and we go through the exercise of taking one thing off, it is most frequently a necklace. The issue is necklace *length*.

Necklaces are too often worn at the incorrect length, creating an unnecessary horizontal "break" in the line of the body. Beware of the "danger zone"—the area that starts at the bottom of your neck (beneath a choker-style necklace) and extends to the top of your cleavage. Avoid little chains or drop pendants or stones that hit your neck in this danger zone. A necklace resting here tends to "break you off" at the neck.

Instead, try one of the two extremes, which I have

185

found look good on women of size. "Long" works well for us (anywhere between forty-two and seventy-two inches), with about forty-six inches looking the best on most women. Long strands of pearls or chains mixed together and worn in multiples create impact. Try wearing two or three together (or even four or five if you want!), combining faux pearls with gold chains and mixes of brightly colored stones. The effect is rich and sumptuous!

Long necklaces tend to draw the eye vertically, up and down the body, giving the illusion of length instead of width. If, however, you have a very large chest, long may not be the best choice, because long chains have to travel *outward* over the line of the bosom and sometimes stick out awkwardly. If you are well endowed in this area, choose necklaces that hit just at the top of the cleavage (between twenty-eight and thirty inches). This will draw the eye upward and sweep it beyond the bosom and the danger zone.

The other extreme that works well on women of size is the choker. Necklaces worn choker style can create an elegant look, particularly for dressy or evening occasions. Contrary to popular belief, chokers do not have to choke you, nor do you have to have an Audrey Hepburn swan neck to wear one. Look at Barbara Bush, for instance. She is a beautiful woman of size, and she regularly (for both day and evening) wears a loose triple-strand choker made by costume jeweler Kenneth Jay Lane. (See Resources.)

A choker necklace immediately draws the attention upward to a beautiful smiling face. However, chokers are not for everyone. How do you know? Try one and see. The test is when you look in the mirror. If a choker is right for you, you will look *comfortable* wearing it. No bulkiness, no strangulation. If it is *not* the right necklace choice, you will see it immediately as you look at yourself in the mirror. Take it off and try a looser version. If it still looks awkward or bulky, then chokers aren't your thing.

Necklaces are the easiest type of jewelry to have made in custom sizes. Chains of all sizes and type are available to purchase in custom lengths. Look for those large "spools" in jewelry stores wound with miles and miles of chain. You decide which style and length you want and they cut it off for you and attach the proper clasp. Instant custom-length necklaces!

Remember impact and scale. If a necklace cannot be seen from twenty paces, ask yourself if it has the correct proportions for your body. And remember, often the *best* neck is a *bare* neck.

Pins are the most underused fashion accessory. Pins were extremely popular during the 1940s and '50s, but since then, they seem to have fallen out of mainstream fashion accessorizing. What a shame! A single but substantial pin or grouping of smaller pins can have more impact and style than any other single jewelry item. Real or costume, pins offer a touch of drama that can change an outfit from "okay" to "magnificent."

A pin brings focus to the face without "cutting" the body at any one spot (as a necklace tends to do.) Pins can evoke the feeling of whimsy and delight, as if a butterfly or flower has landed on top of your shoulder. Pins can also offer an understated elegance if you choose to wear a bejeweled Maltese cross or a rhinestone feather or crown pin. These classic motifs are always in style and can be found in many styles and designs.

There's one trick to pin wearing and here it is. If you are going to wear a pin on your shoulder, it should always be worn *high*—almost on top of the shoulder—attracting attention *upward* toward the face. The focus should be

187

up, up, up, broadening the horizon and illuminating the face. Whenever I work with a woman who is wearing a pin on her lapel, I ask her to try it higher on her shoulder. There is an immediate difference in the dramatic touch it brings by moving it upward to the *top* of the shoulder. A good rule of thumb is to avoid wearing pins anywhere below your collarbone. Higher is better.

A pin can be worn in "surprise" spots as well . . . perhaps two or three small jeweled snails climbing up the sleeve of a simple long-sleeved dress or a rhinestone bee at the lowest point of a simple black dress with a plunging back. Another "surprise spot" is dead center at the lowest point of a V-neck blouse or dress. A daring Texas socialite wears her Cartier panther pin crawling down the décolletage of a V-neck blouse. A little racy, yes, but the idea here is to practice creativity with your pins. Try clustering several of the same type together.

Dig out your old pins and see if they work with any of your clothes. If not, clear the clutter by giving them to someone who can use them, and start over by collecting one or two great pins to add to your look!

As women of size, we have to be cautious about wearing bracelets, or any wrist adornment for that matter. All too often jewelry on the wrists can make our arms appear shorter and our hands look out of proportion to the rest of our body. Worn correctly, however, by adhering to several tips, bracelets can be a great fashion accessory for women of size.

The first rule to remember about bracelets is that *fit is everything.* Nothing is more unattractive than a bracelet that is too small, squeezing and biting into the flesh of the wrist. Bracelets should be worn loose and comfortable (with the exception of "cuffs").

I have discovered in my years of living inside a larger body that many of the bracelets available (especially costume jewelry) are too small. This calls for a little bit of patience and ingenuity. Patience because it takes patience to keep searching far and wide for bracelets that fit. My advice here is to keep trying. There is no one "standard" size in bracelets. The range can be anywhere from six to nine inches, depending on the style. I have found that bracelets made of natural materials such as wood or bamboo tend to be larger because they are usually made by hand instead of by a machine.

The search takes ingenuity because we have to think creatively to create new solutions for our wrist-size challenges. Put two bracelets together to make one that fits. Buy a necklace and break it down into two or three bracelets. Make your own bracelet out of beads and fishing wire. Have your jeweler expand bracelets with extra links. I was once given an expensive thick silver cuff bracelet that was too small to go around my wrist. I took it to the jeweler and he slowly heated the silver until it was malleable, then he stretched it to my exact wrist size.

I have also discovered a lifesaver called a jewelry extender, a small extension clip and ring that instantly loosens tight bracelets. Jewelry extenders are available in 24k gold plate and sterling silver plate in three sizes: small ($\frac{1}{2}$ inch), medium ($\frac{3}{4}$ inch), and large ($1\frac{1}{2}$ inches). (See Resources.)

Your bracelets should remain bold and simple. Cuff bracelets work on very few women. Unless you have long, super-skinny arms, they tend to give a chopped-off effect. Charm bracelets are good. Just make sure you have added extra links to the length of the bracelet over the years so that you have a proper fit. A bracelet should be loose

enough to turn easily in circles around your wrist but not
so loose as to slide off your hand.

How about watches? Some women have no interest
in wristwatches and others don't dream of walking out
the door without one. If you wear a watch, here are a few
handy reminders for well-rounded women.

I recommend owning one simple, classic all-around
watch for everyday wear and a durable sports watch. If
you can afford it, spend your money on a great-looking
everyday watch. Simple means no diamonds, no ornate
designs or bands. There are a multitude of watches to
choose from in everyone's price range—from a Cartier
"Tank" watch (around $2,500) to an understated Timex
from the drugstore (around $30).

Your second watch should be a "knock-around"
watch for tennis, yard work, days at the beach. I use a
good-looking men's watch worn as a sports watch. You
can get a version of a classic men's "diving watch" for as
little as $75 (try to find one with the fewest gauges and
gadgets . . . unless you are a diver!). Inexpensive, simple
Swatch watches make great sports watches. Try to find
one that has a clean face void of cartoons or clever say-
ings. Think *simple, functional, classic.* A friend of mine
(who has more than enough money to own any watch in
the world) wears a simple Swatch with a white face, black
numbers, and a black band. I wear a men's Timex as my
knock-around watch. It's big, has a simple face and design, and the price was right.

A note on "evening" or "dressy occasion" watches. I
don't own one because I do not like the look of a watch
(any watch) worn with evening clothes. To me, its very
presence insults the festivity of a special event or party.
A watch on a woman in formal (or even cocktail) attire,
denotes that she is mindful of the time—something I
don't think is an attractive party look. A dressy party is

not a business meeting, it is time meant for revelry making, not clock watching. If you feel you must have some sort of timepiece, I recommend keeping a small watch face on a black satin ribbon tied inside your evening bag. Any old watch face will do, just remove the band and thread it onto a satin ribbon tied off at both ends. If you feel you must know what time it is you can open your evening bag, follow the black ribbon with your fingers, and sneak a look at the watch face.

How to choose a watch size? Again, scale and fit are everything. Scale: in general, a watch with a larger face is more attractive for women of size. It will also be easier for you to read. A smaller watch will look out of proportion with the rest of your body. Don't forget to try the men's department when you shop for your watch. The scale is bigger and generally better for women of size.

Fit: a watch that is too tight looks cheap and shabby, not to mention *uncomfortable*. I have had the band changed on practically every watch I have ever owned. For as little as $12, you can have a new leather band that fits. Again, try using men's bands instead of women's because they are bigger and better looking. As far as metal link bands are concerned, you can always take your watch to the jeweler and have more links added.

Rings draw attention and focus to your hands. If you don't consider your hands as one of your positives, I would forget about rings altogether. Unadorned hands are less noticeable, and allow the focus to be diverted elsewhere. If you do choose to wear rings, here are a few guidelines to help you choose the right rings.

Wear only *one* or *two* rings at a time. Don't overdo it. Too many rings lose their impact and look gaudy and cheap. If you wear a wedding and engagement ring on your left ring finger, keep it simple and avoid wearing

191

other rings. However, if you feel you *must* wear another ring, make *sure* it's on the other hand. And please, no rings on index fingers or thumbs. I have yet to see a woman who looks attractive with a ring on either of these fingers.

When buying rings, try them on late in the day, when your fingers are the most swollen from the natural day's activities. This way you are sure to get a ring that won't become tight and uncomfortable by day's end. I have always had to have my rings sized to fit. Very rarely, perhaps never, have I walked up to a jewelry counter and found a ring that fit right off the bat. Sizing up is not a big deal, and it will allow you to actually *wear* those rings that are sitting dormant (and two sizes too small) in your jewelry box.

Remember the concept of *impact* when choosing rings. Forgo the microscopic diamond chips in favor of larger semiprecious stones or a big gold or silver dome ring. And if there is any doubt about whether a ring is right or not, it probably *isn't.* Rings are not for everyone. Rings actually shorten the perceived length of our fingers. Decide if you have fingers on which rings are flattering.

If you do decide that rings are your thing, always, but *always,* keep your hands well manicured and clean. Remember, rings only draw attention to the hands and fingers, and no one wants to call attention to chipped polish or ragged cuticles. Keep your hands and nails in great shape and wear your rings with pride.

Scarves

I adore scarves. There is no quicker way to change the look of your uniform(s) than with a well-chosen scarf. Scarves add a punch of color and a hint of movement which can pick up an otherwise ordinary outfit.

There are many types of scarves to choose from, but the main thing to keep in mind is size! Women of size need bigger scarves. The most prevalent scarf size in stores today is the traditional thirty-six-inch square (such as the classic Hermès silk scarves), which is not big enough for us. It is just too little fabric to create any sort of impact on the scale of our bodies. A folded thirty-six-inch scarf barely goes round my neck once, and leaves *nothing* to drape, fall, or flow.

Small square scarves look chintzy, boring, and cheap. Scarves are meant to be dramatic and bold, creating a sense of movement and flow on the body. I do own several thirty-six-inch scarves (most were given to me as gifts) and I can suggest several ways to utilize the small scarves you may already own.

1. Wear it over your head à la Grace Kelly. Fold into a triangle and crisscross the ends under your chin and tie at the back of your neck. Add big sunglasses and you have instant glamour.
2. Tie it to the handles of your purse in a secure square knot (right over left, left over right) and let it add a dash of color and interest to your pocketbook or tote bag.
3. Use it as a jacket lapel "liner." Put the scarf around your neck, untied, and wear it between a blouse and jacket, with the ends untethered but securely tucked or pinned inside. (You must plan to keep your jacket on to do this.) Tuck the ends vertically along the inside of the jacket lapel, allowing just a hint of the scarf to mimic the lines of lapel. The scarf will add a punch of color to the outfit, and no one will know how small the scarf really is since it is tucked in and the jacket stays on.

4. Have your beautiful silk thirty-six-inch scarves cut down to squares twelve by twelve inches (with finished edges) and give them to your favorite gentleman who is a snappy dresser, to use as pocket squares.

5. And now the most extravagant of all! I know a girl in New York who "grew out" of her thirty-six-inch square Hermès silk scarf collection. (She quit her nine-to-five Wall Street job where "yuppies" in thirty-six-inch scarves *thrive!*) Instead of letting her scads and scads of silk scarves sit in the drawer, she had them all sewn together patchwork style into a stunning set of colorful, chic curtains for her dressing room. Extravagant? Yes. But I love it, don't you? You could achieve the same sort of effect by having throw pillows made from your scarves.

We have established that thirty-six-inch scarves don't work on bigger bodies. So what's the answer? The answer is a big square scarf measuring at least fifty inches square or an oversized oblong scarf somewhere along the lines of 108 by 40 inches. In my consulting work, women often ask me how to "tie" their scarves. My answer to them is that once you start wearing scarves that are big enough, you don't have to worry about how to tie them. Tying is no longer the issue. If you have enough material to work with, you can basically tie it any way you please and it will come out looking great. Leave all those silly scarf-tying tricks to the uninformed women still wearing those tiny thirty-six-inch squares. When you have a big enough piece of material to work with, draping, tying and arranging is simplified. You won't need fancy knots or tricks. Throw it on and go!

Big squares are the perfect size for us because they actually reach all the way around ample shoulders and have room left to tie off. My fifty-four-inch square scarf is even long enough to wear folded as a belt. Big square scarves can be found in many different fabrics. See if you can find one in wool or a wool and cashmere blend to wear on the *outside* of a classic overcoat or trench. You can use a big, simple pin or clip to hold the scarf in place. (Remember, even scarf pins still go *high, high, high* on the shoulder!)

Oblong scarves are also real winners. Please make sure they are long enough. I think any length ninety inches or longer is sufficient because it gives you enough fabric to play with. Oblongs look terrific looped behind the neck once and tied in a loose, low knot in front, hanging free and creating an elongated V shape. Or, just the opposite . . . make the loop in front of your neck and let the ends hang and float free behind you. Choose a sheer chiffon scarf for this look—it makes for a dramatic entrance (or exit!).

If you have trouble finding oblong scarves that are long enough, don't worry. Oblongs are the easiest to make. Most fabrics sold in fabric stores come in widths of thirty-six to forty-two inches. When you choose a fabric, think in advance about which fabrics drape and tie the best. Choose a beautiful chiffon or silk and have two and a half yards cut (ninety inches). Have the two ends and the two sides finished to prevent fraying, and voilà! You have your custom-made oblong scarf ready to wear. Once I found a thirty-six-inch square scarf that I adored. Knowing full well that there was no way I could wear a scarf that small, I bought three of them and had them sewn together end to end to make one long scarf 108 by 36 inches. (Do this only with scarves whose designs are busy enough that the seams won't show.)

Big scarves are multifunctional. Have a big square cotton scarf for summer. Wrap it around your hips as a sarong to the beach, and then take it off and use it as you would a beach towel! Collect big scarves in cashmere or wool for winter. Use them as a wrap on those not-cold-enough-for-a-coat evenings. I own a ninety-six-inch black cashmere "scarf" that I use as an evening shawl; as a day-time wrap over leggings; as a long scarf over my coat on cold, cold days; and as my snuggly blanket on long air-plane trips. It's been worth the price I paid for it since it fulfills so many needs!

Belts

As women of size, we either look good in belts or we do not. It's usually one or the other, with no in betweens. Generally speaking (and from the experience of working with hundreds of women,) belts work best on bodies that have some waist definition. In other words, if your waist measurement is six to eight inches smaller than your hips, you have a better chance of wearing belts well. If belts do not mesh with your body type or your uniform needs, *forget them* and move on. Although a belt can be an interesting and eye-catching fashion accessory, one must always keep in mind that belts create a strong horizontal line across the midsection of your body.

First, decide exactly what you will be wearing the belt with. Jeans? Slacks? A dress or a skirt? I recommend matching the belt color to the color of the garment you plan to wear it with. In other words, if you need a belt for a long denim skirt, choose one that is predominately navy or some shade of blue. For black trousers, you would want a good black leather or black suede belt. By matching colors you achieve the maximum interest a belt can provide with a minimum of attention drawn to the horizontal line it creates.

When trying on belts, move around, bend over, and sit down. Be sure that the belt does not fold over on itself when you sit. It should rest comfortably with all your movements. Certain care should be taken to choose the belt that is best for you, knowing that you only need to own a few, good belts in basic, neutral colors.

Neutral-color belts are the most versatile and easiest to find. Black, dark brown, saddle leather, and navy are the neutrals that make up a basic belt wardrobe. Avoid plastic belts. They tend to crack or peel and they hold more heat, making you sweaty at the belt line. Don't ever wear a belt that you can buckle only on the last notch. It just looks *bad.*

Chain belts are okay as long as they are big enough to drape and swag around the waist and hips instead of fitting too closely. If a single chain belt doesn't offer enough length to work with, buy two or three and put them together, looping them around your waist several times to create more impact. Gold chain-link belts should be worn low, sort of slung or swagged across the top of the hip line—not tight at the waist.

If you cannot find good leather belts in your size, how about having one made? Many shoe repair and leather shops will make any belt you want in any length. Bring your own buckle, preferably a gold or silver-plated one in a simple design, pick a leather you like (have it dyed if need be), and you will have created your own custom-made belt.

Hats and Gloves

Hats can add the all-important touch of drama to your wardrobe. Well-rounded women are made to wear hats! In fact, we generally wear hats better than many of our smaller sisters. The scale and generous proportions of our bodies can carry off the drama and flair associated with hats. The trick to wearing a hat well is to wear it with *confidence.* When trying on hats, use this general rule of thumb: If it *feels* silly, then chances are it probably looks silly. If it *feels* good, then it more than likely looks good.

Stylishness aside, hats are the most practical fashion accessories you can own. In the winter wear hats to preserve body heat, as we lose 75 percent of it through the top of the head. In the summer, hats shield us from the sun's direct rays and keep the head cool. If you are new to hat wearing, start by thinking practically. You will want a hat for winter, one for summer, and perhaps a rain hat.

For winter, think warmth. *Any* hat, even a baseball cap (which I do not recommend unless you are exercising or playing a sport), will significantly decrease the loss of body heat through your head. Knitted caps are great for warmth when you are skiing but fall short in the style department for everyday wear. Try different styles, maybe a wool fedora or beret. Decide whether you look better in a large brim or a smaller one. The taller you are, the larger the brim can be. Don't buy a hat that you would be afraid to expose to the rain, sleet, or snow. Winter hats have a job to do even while they are enhancing your look.

For the summer, you will want to look for a hat to provide shade for your face and neck. I like big straw hats and have several shapes and styles that I wear all summer long. If you buy one good straw hat, you can change the look by switching the hat band using a strip of different-colored grosgrain, linen, or cotton madras. Straw hats or hats of a natural weave are most suitable for summer because they provide shade for the face yet allow the head to aerate or breathe through the open weave.

Gloves, too, can be functional items in your accessory wardrobe. Make sure you have several pairs for wintertime warmth in assorted colors and fabrics. You can have fun with gloves. Brighten a cold winter's day by wearing lipstick-red gloves. For added warmth be sure to buy gloves lined in silk or cashmere.

Here's a wonderful styling trick I learned from years of modeling. Gloves are just as useful as a fashion accessory once you are *inside* and have taken them off. Do you ever feel awkward with your hands? Gloves are the perfect solution for not knowing what to do with your hands. Instead of tucking gloves away in your purse or coat pocket, carry them neatly folded together in one hand. Gloves can keep your hands occupied, punctuating your conversation and accentuating your hand movements.

Shoes

Wearing the right pair of shoes is important for women of size for two reasons. First, shoes are a visible telltale sign of our fashion finesse. Many times you'll see a beautiful plus-size woman dressed to a "T"—but not down to her *toes*. She'll get everything else right and then throw on a ratty old pair of shoes. Nothing kills a look faster than bad shoes. Secondly, all of our body weight ends up carried around on our feet. As well-rounded women, we need to be extra mindful that we are getting the proper support from our shoes.

Have a plan for your shoes much as you do for your clothes. Begin by throwing away all the old shoes that you have never worn because you bought them a half size too small. Next, get rid of any shoes that are in extremely poor repair. Grubby, worn-out shoes are, from this point forward, forever banished from your wardrobe.

Now decide which types of shoes work best with each of your uniforms and make a concise list of your shoe needs. Remember to keep it basic and simple. In order to create a basic shoe wardrobe, you should initially stick to neutral shoes that can service a variety of footwear needs.

Comfort is everything. In order to get comfort, you have to buy well-made shoes. Although they cost more, well-made shoes last longer. Find a brand of shoe that fits you well and stick to it. I have the curse *and* the blessing of wearing a size 11 shoe. It is a curse because there is, comparatively speaking, very little available in anything over size 10. It is a blessing because I was forced to wear Ferragamo shoes (a venerable Italian shoe designer known for quality and comfort) from a very early age because that was the only line of shoes available in size 11. When all of my friends in junior high were wearing the latest mod "platform" shoes, I wore sensible, black, Italian leather, low-heeled shoes with the classic Ferragamo bow on the toe. From that time on, I have been addicted to shoes that are made for support *and* comfort. Find a shoe make that offers a variety of style options and gives you the support you need. Now some more quick shoe tips.

1. You decide if high heels are right for you. Some women like them, some women hate them. It's pretty much up to you and your personal preference. However, even a smallish heel (one to two inches) elongates the line of the leg, creating a more graceful silhouette. Do not wear high heels if you are not comfortable doing so—it creates an unnatural gait and signals to the world that you are uneasy and uncomfortable.

2. Take care of your shoes. Don't let your shoes get scruffy or worn down. Keep your shoes in top form—no holes in the soles, no ragged-looking heels, no missing or worn-down heel tips. That unbearable "click, click, click" sound when the rubber (or plastic) heel tip is worn off and you are walking around on the nail head is the all-time worst shoe-maintenance faux pas. Keep a little shoe repair kit at home complete with soft rag, shoe polish, and a suede brush to take care of all minor touch-ups. Find a shoe repair shop where they can take care of the rest of your shoe maintenance needs.

3. Invest in rubber soles for all your good leather shoes. Before I wear a pair of new shoes for the first time, I take them to the cobbler, and for around $20, I have a thin rubber sole glued to the bottom all my shoes. This is a must if you are as hard on your shoes as I am on mine, because it prevents the sole from wearing out. The rubber sole will *triple* the life of the shoes.

4. Unless you have shapely ankles that you want to call attention to, avoid ankle straps. They cut the line of the leg at the ankle and make legs look larger and shorter.

5. Keep your shoes simple. Less is definitely more when it comes to shoes. Shoes should be understated and go basically unnoticed. Your choice of footwear should remain cohesive with the rest of your look. Wearing a well-made shoe of simple design is the most attractive statement a woman can make.

6. If you wear open-toe shoes or sandals, be sure your feet are in show-off shape. That means *clean, groomed, and pedicured.*

7. Don't wear sneakers to the office. I understand why so many women do it. I know they change into their

"work shoes" the minute they get to the office. It still doesn't make it right. There are shoes available today that are constructed for walking and have the look of an "office shoe." Save sneakers for the weekends.

Handbags/Purses

A few good bags are all you need. Purses are fashion necessities that can easily be pared down to the barest of chic, functional minimums. Our lives are too busy to afford the luxury (if not headache) of having a bag to match every outfit. In fact, the only women I know who coordinate a bag for every outfit are Queen Elizabeth and the Queen Mother. It's a charming thought, but most of us do not have the time to afford such a luxury. Your purse should be well made and sturdy, offering flexibility to adapt to a variety of looks.

You must start with two good-quality everyday bags—one for fall and winter and one for spring and summer. These will be the mainstays of your purse wardrobe. Decide which *size* purse works best to fit your lifestyle and search out a well-made leather bag. Think longevity. Save up to purchase something that you will use for *years,* not months. Imagine yourself pulling this same purse out year after year and having it fit beautifully into your wardrobe.

For the summer months, you can afford to have several woven straw bags in your purse wardrobe. They are inexpensive and functional, and although you may not want to carry them to the office (unless they are a tight, neat weave), straw bags are a welcome summertime fashion accessory.

The other staple in your handbag wardrobe should be an evening bag. I actually advise my clients to own two; one black and one neutral metallic. These two options should carry you through any and every evening event from a cocktail party to a black-tie ball. Keep them simple in design and free of too much detail, so that they are certain to offer maximum versatility.

Purse-buying hints for women of size:

1. Size: decide what size looks best on your body by standing before a full-length mirror and trying several different sizes and styles. Not every size looks good on every body. If big bags overpower you, stick to compact smaller sizes. If a small bag gets lost on your frame, try a larger one. Trust the mirror to tell you which size is best for your body and your needs. If your purse is always stuffed and "busting at the seams" (a very unattractive state of affairs), you need to buy a larger bag. Likewise, you don't want to carry such large bags that you look like a pack mule. Try different sizes and see what works best for you.

2. Focus. Your purse or tote bag will draw focus to the exact location where it hits your body. Make sure you *plan* where you want the focus to be. For example, I have to have a shoulder bag that hits me high, resting just under my armpit, or low, resting well below my hip line. Bags that hit me anywhere near my midsection tend to draw extra, unwanted attention to my middle area and tummy. If you want your purse to draw attention away from your body, choose a purse with handles that you can carry by hand or around your wrist.

3. Accessibility: my friend Malissa once owned an expensive designer purse that her mother gave her. Although it was very beautiful, she called it the "Cave" because it was dark and cavernous and had a very

small opening—fine for a cave but not for a purse. She was *forever* digging around in the Cave, groping and hoping to pull out whatever item she was looking for.

Your bag must have easy accessibility. No matter how attractive a purse might be, it must function to help your day-to-day activities, rather than hinder them. Women of size are sometimes unjustly accused of being lazy or unorganized. Keeping one's things in order (even in your purse) offsets this stereotype and promotes the image of calm efficiency.

Really *look* inside a purse before you purchase it. How well can you see inside? Is the opening big enough for your wallet? Take out the tissue paper and try putting all your things in it. Does everything fit? Check out the accessibility factor *before* you buy.

4. Color is a personal preference. However, when buying a purse, it is advisable to stick to the neutral tones for several reasons. Dark neutrals such as burgundy, black, dark brown, saddle brown, and navy offer the most versatility season to season—saving money and time. Instead of owning many different-colored bags to match every outfit, you can easily adapt a few neutral bags to many different looks and color palettes. Neutral colors also "age" the best because they tend to show less wear and tear over time. As women of size, we want to be noticed for the overall picture we present, rather than for a loud, showy bag or purse.

And to close, a word about "fanny packs." I don't care what size you wear, belted fanny packs are one of the most unattractive accessories ever invented. I believe that they should be reserved for the sport of hiking, and hiking only. These pouches destroy the line of anything you are wearing and only draw attention to your lower body—your hips, thighs, and stomach. Opt for a fashionable backpack if you must have your arms free of a purse or tote bag. Backpacks can be slung casually (and vertically) over a shoulder, which is much more attractive than a huge horizontal pouch slung across the middle of your body.

The Scale of Your Life: Life Accessories

Scale and proportion do not stop at our fashion accessories. For women of size, scale and proportion affect every area of our lives—every space we inhabit and everything we touch. "Life accessories" are those elements that come into play in our lives *outside* of what we wear. Life accessories are to be found in our immediate surroundings—a chair, a desk, a glass, a car, a pillow, an arrangement of flowers. Most people don't even think about the scale or proportion of such elements, leaving their presence in life to chance and fate.

As a well-rounded woman, I have found, however, that life accessories *can work to our advantage* when we can adapt them to the laws of scale and proportion appropriate for *our* bodies. Because we have the privilege of occupying more space in the world, we need to be mindful of how we come into contact with the landscape of our lives.

Let me give you several examples to explain. One of the most obvious life accessories is furniture. When you walk into a party do you take a moment to decide *where* you will sit? *Where* you will be most comfortable and in which chair you will be able to maximize your assets?

I have taught myself to walk into a room, a restau-

205

rant, or office and quickly "size up" the furniture. I first eliminate any seating that does not look sturdy enough to hold me. There's no use sitting in a rickety chair and worrying that it will collapse at any moment. I then rule out any big, mushy, cushy sofas or chairs, knowing I won't look my best climbing into or out of them. I usually try to spot a sturdy armchair with a straight back. Once, at a dinner party, I even asked the hostess if I could move a chair from another room into the room where we are sitting (I blamed it on a bad back!). You will find that people are more than willing to comply with your special requests as long as you ask for them with smile.

Check out the furniture in your own house. Does it serve you and your body well? Is it both comfortable *and* functional? Make sure that you don't own furniture that you cannot or will not use. Much of the "antique" furniture sold today was designed and made in the nineteenth century, when people were smaller. In fact, in the 1800s, the average man stood five feet, six inches, and women were even smaller than that. Picture in your mind's eye how you would look in a chair before you sit it. In your own house, opt for a few pieces of attractive, well-made furniture with ample size and scale that will last for years.

Other life accessories to think about are everyday items such as the wineglasses you own. Do they have the correct scale and proportion to flatter your hand when you hold them or do they look minuscule and oddly out of proportion with the rest of your body as you hold them? It's your house, your stage. You might as well set the stage for your comfort and for you to look your best!

Is your car roomy enough for you to move and drive comfortably? I know cars are a big-ticket item, but again, owning and enjoying a car that is the right size for your body to function in is just another way of accepting and celebrating your real-life accessories. Take a moment to think of all the "things" that you come into contact with every day. Try to gauge if they are in proper scale and proportion to your body. Are they comfortable for your well-rounded body and life? Are you compromising your comfort in any way? You will find that with a little thought along these lines, there are many things that we can control or adjust to fit and complement our well-rounded bodies.

Exceptions to Scale and Proportion Rules

Now that I've just told you to adapt your life accessories to fit your body, I have to give you the *exceptions* to the rule! Food and men don't count when it comes to scale, proportion, or size. Let me explain.

The first is food. My general rule of thumb is eat what you want, when you want it, in front of whomever you wish. It breaks my heart to see women of size in restaurants ordering "a small green salad with dressing on the side" for the main course of their dinner because they worry what others will think if they just eat a normal, healthy, delicious meal. I mean, we aren't fooling anyone. Everyone can see our luscious curves—so why pretend that we only want a salad? I think it is attractive to have a healthy appetite—an interest in good food and a lusty, unparsimonious attitude about eating.

Conversely, I do not recommend eating enormous amounts of food either. Eat (not overeat) when you are hungry, stop when you are almost full. As simple as it sounds, this is the oldest food rule around. Don't be shy about stating your food needs and/or desires (see more about food in the next step).

The important thing is to smile, laugh, drink, eat, and enjoy with others. So often women of size work their way into "closet" eating—eating alone and in private for fear someone will make comment. Learn to have a healthy attitude about the food you eat. Don't be embarrassed to ask for seconds—but also know how to stop when you have had enough. Break bread with friends and loved ones, appreciating the bounty of food available and how it nourishes your beautiful body!

As for loved ones—your husband, boyfriend, man, significant other, or life partner—they don't have to be any certain size to be a perfect fit for you. I am writing this because many women (my best friend and my mother, for example) feel that their partner has to be bigger and taller than they are. Balderdash! I mean, we all have our personal preferences, but great things can come in small packages!

A woman once told me that she couldn't go out with a guy who wore smaller jeans than she did. As women of size, if we ruled out every guy who wore jeans smaller than ours, we'd be cutting out hundreds of thousands of interesting people. It is size discrimination in reverse! Here's a secret. The sexiest man I ever went out with was *half* my size.

P.S. I bet professional model Jerry Hall can't fit into her husband's jeans . . . she's a curvaceous six-foot-tall Texan, and Mick Jagger is only five feet, eight inches!

Accessorizing your life means learning how to see your beautiful well-rounded body in relation to everything around it. Don't shy away from your glorious space. You have it, you might as well use it, cherish it, adorn it, and celebrate it in every way you can to embody the new well-rounded you.

1. Make one or several *nonbuying* trips to your favorite department store to try, test, and play with different size and scale fashion accessories, including jewelry, scarves, belts, hats and gloves, shoes, and purses. Make this a fact-finding venture—gathering information on the size, scale, and proportion of fashion accessories so they look best on you.

2. Decide on one fashion accessory that you could easily adopt as a signature accessory. Pull it out, dust it off, and make it your trademark.

3. Reassess your existing fashion accessories. Keep only the ones that you use, that fit, and have the correct scale and proportion for your body. Give the rest away.

4. Open up your awareness to the life accessories around you. Notice how proportionate they are to your body and if they are scaled to complement your life.

What wondrous life is
this I lead!
Ripe apples drop about my head;
The luscious clusters of the vine
Upon my mouth do crush their wine;
The nectarine, and curious peach,
Into my hands themselves do reach;
Stumbling on melons, as I pass,
Ensnared with flowers,
I fall on grass.

—ANDREW MARVELL

Evaluate Your Relationship with Food

No matter what we do or where we go, we will always have to eat. Food keeps us alive. It gives us the energy and nourishment we need to live. Food will always be part of our lives. We all have some sort of relationship with food. Most of us have deep-rooted feelings about it—some positive and some negative. I am still learning about food. I work every day to create and maintain a harmonious, loving, and healthy relationship with food. It isn't always easy.

Food is everywhere. Food will not go away. You cannot sweep it under the carpet or lock it up in a closet. It will always be part of your life. I tried for many years to "give up" my feelings for food—negating its importance and trying desperately to "forget about it," "ignore it," or even "hate it." It never worked. For years I would say that I wished I didn't have to deal with food at all. I fantasized about a "food pill" that would alleviate the need to ever eat again. Alas, there is no such pill.

When I went on a medically supervised fast for five months, I thought I had finally found a way to ignore food. I simply *gave it up*—drinking a powder-and-water mixture instead. During the fast, I didn't have to make any decisions about what to eat, when to eat, or how much to eat. It was all wonderful until I had to reintroduce food into my life at the end of the fast. I had lost weight, but hadn't gained any of the tools or information I needed to deal with food on a daily basis.

When the fast was over, I was face-to-face with food

again—more confused than ever and eating my way back up the scale. Giving up food doesn't work. We have to search and find a new *respect* for food—*face it* and *make peace* with it. It is then we begin to understand food as our *ally*, not our enemy.

It's only natural that we think about food often. We have lived through so many negative dieting experiences where food has been unnaturally rationed, portioned, and even denied altogether, that the very topic of food has become a hotbed of swirling, confused emotions. Food is a big issue in our lives. Let's face it. It's been a big issue for us for many, many years, and it is difficult to just turn off all those emotions we have about it. The emotions are deep rooted from years of dieting and losing and gaining weight, weighing ourselves obsessively and adopting unnatural eating habits. The fact that we *think* about food is not going to change.

What *can* change are the very thoughts we have about food. My thinking about food changed from hate to love. From dependence to peaceful coexistence. And from fear to respect. This happened little by little over a period of years. It happened by *relaxing* and listening to my body—using common sense and refusing to "diet" ever again. By doing these things, I was able to alleviate my anxiety about food and concentrate on a new relationship. I took the pressure off myself and decided to get comfortable with my food. I made the decision to allow food to work *with* me instead of *against* me.

The relationship I enjoy with food these days is one based on trust and respect. I *trust* that my body will tell me what it needs and when. I *trust* in my decision to never go on a "diet" again. I *respect* food and the ability it has to make my body function so efficiently. Let me show you how to begin your own new relationship with food.

Give Up Dieting Forever:
A Personalized Approach

You tell me. Dieting doesn't work, does it? Smile, relax, say adios, and move on to a new relationship with your food based on trust, respect, and understanding.

Everyone's food needs are different. The way *you* need to eat is completely exclusive to *you* and *your body's* chemistry. Throughout my lifetime, nutrition has been based around hard, unyielding lines. *Daily requirements, dietary requirements, balanced meals,* and *recommended daily allowances* are phrases that we all grew up with, and they're still around today even though they are beginning to sound increasingly archaic.

Thankfully, modern nutrition is slowly starting to accept that there is more than *one* right way to eat, *one* right food pyramid to follow, and more than *one* right number of calories to consume. We are moving into a time when people are becoming more in tune with their *own bodies* and their *own individual food needs.* "The norm," "the standard," "the average," and "the recommended" are becoming obsolete, and we are beginning to understand that there is no right or wrong way to approach food. There is no such thing as a *normal* diet, a *standard* size portion, an *average* number of calories or *recommended* daily allowance.

Many factors contribute to the wide variety of eating habits. First, we all have different lifestyles and ways of eating to properly accommodate them. We eat when, where, and how we do to try to maximize our "output" and sustain our energy level throughout the day. Second, we each have different dietary needs. My body doesn't tolerate dairy products well; yours may crave them. Our eating reflects our unique dietary needs. Third, we are each biologically and genetically programmed to gravitate toward the types of foods that we need to sustain us. This is based on our ethnic background and what and where our ancestors ate throughout the centuries.

Nutrition, or just plain old *eating,* is a very personal issue. There is no single, universally correct way to eat. It is essential to create our own *personal eating plan* based on our *unique* body and its *specific* needs. Stop thinking about *which diet to follow.* Instead, begin to listen to the signals your body is giving you and, around those needs, build a personalized food plan just for you!

Listen to Your Body

Your body has an intelligence all its own. It knows exactly what type of food it needs, how much it needs, and when it needs it. Your body is a perfectly functioning machine. It will let you know what it requires by sending internal "signals" to you. The challenge here is to be able to *hear* the signals your body is giving you.

By "signals" I am referring to the internal *longings* you get for a certain type of food, or a feeling inside that tells you that you are very hungry. For example, I know that if I don't eat some sort of protein before the early afternoon, I will experience a mild headache. The headache is a signal from my body telling me that it is time to eat a protein such as meat, eggs, fish, or cheese. When I do, the headache goes away.

Our signals become very clear on days when we are busy and put off eating until later than usual. We start to feel tired and sluggish, unable to perform even the most simple task until we give our body the fuel it needs. Fatigue is a signal that your body is giving you, telling you to eat. You will also feel tired if you are not eating all the nutrients that your body needs. The fatigue is your body's way of telling you, "What you just fed me didn't work. . . . I didn't need a [carbohydrate]. I need a [protein]." If you want the fatigue to go away, you must experiment with foods and find the ones that make your body feel *alive* and *energetic,* rather than tired and slow.

Over the years and through constant dieting, we lose the ability to hear our own internal body signals. Dieting causes the signals to become blocked. The endless cycles of lose-and-gain, gain-and-lose, along with constant food denial and deprivation, have conditioned us to "tune out" our natural body signals. By refusing our bodies food while on a diet, we learn to ignore the natural hunger signals our bodies give us. By bingeing or eating too much at any given time we cause the signals to become "muffled" and repressed. The result of all this is that we can never really "hear" what our body wants or needs.

So what's the answer? How do you begin listening to your own body signals? *Awareness* is most of it. Just being *aware* that your body is talking to you will help you to hear the signals. Learning to listen takes time. Start slowly and lovingly. To begin, you will want to listen for *when* your body needs food. See if you can accurately discern the times of day (or evening) when your body tells you it truly *needs* food. Once you are able to do this with some regularity, you will begin to hear signals of what *types* of food your body wants. Go slowly. Don't force it. It won't happen overnight. Before I go to sleep at night, I try to remember to thank my body for the signals it gave me all day long. I then ask my body to give me clear food signals the next day as well.

I know, however, that there are other circumstances due to allergies, medications, or other biological concerns that prevent us from clearly hearing our internal signals. Check with your doctor to be sure you are not taking unnecessary medications, or that your needs might dictate a new type or intensity of medication. All of these factors directly relate to how well you can hear your internal body signals.

In my experience, an excess accumulation of "water weight" can significantly distort the degree to which I can "hear" my own internal body signals. To offset this, I cut back on my sodium intake, thus reducing the fluid retention within my body. The less "puffiness" I have due to water retention, the more clearly I can hear my body talking to me and telling me what types of food it needs.

Note: Contrary to popular belief, most of the excess sodium (or salt) that Americans ingest comes *not* from the salt shaker on the table or stove top, but rather from processed foods, fast foods, canned or frozen foods. To successfully reduce your intake of sodium, switch to fresh foods instead of processed foods.

Strive to Eat More Fresh Foods

The switch to fresh foods is one you'll never regret. By increasing your intake of fresh fruits and vegetables you can boost your energy level, clear your skin, and ensure complete and efficient cleansing of your system. ("*Green* inside is *clean* inside!")

Try to make the switch away from convenience foods or any pre-prepared food items. Generally speaking, nonfresh foods (foods with added chemicals) are loaded with sodium and fat, which enhance the taste and act as preservatives to prolong their shelf life. A good rule of thumb for deciding whether or not you should eat a prepared food is to read first the ingredients on the label. If you cannot pronounce one or more of the listed ingredients, think twice about putting it into your body.

Instead, see how close you can come to eating foods that are "straight from the garden," with as little human intervention as possible. Have you ever tasted a yam baked in its natural state *before* you make it into sweet potato pie? It is the most delicious thing in the world. Or how about a fresh fig instead of a Fig Newton? There's no comparison! I generally hear from people that they like prepared foods because they "taste better"—when in fact, they aren't tasting the actual food at all! Once you become accustomed to eating simple, natural foods, processed foods will begin to lose their appeal—tasting too much like the chemicals and additives they contain.

Making small changes to natural foods can make big differences in how your body feels. Try fresh fruit instead of canned or frozen. Make your own tomato sauce instead of buying the canned type. Olive oil, vinegar, lemon juice, a touch of mustard, garlic, and a little salt and pepper make the most delicious homemade salad dressing—much better than anything that comes in a bottle. In fact, lemon juice is a great replacement for salt. If it's flavoring you want, try natural seasonings for your food by using herbs. Basil, rosemary, sage, and parsley are easy to grow in pots and provide delicious, fresh savory or sweet seasonings year-round.

It is recommended that fresh fruits and vegetables should make up 70 percent of what we eat every day. This percentage is not about losing weight. It's about keeping our bodies functioning at their optimal level—ingesting, digesting, and expelling foods that will encourage and maintain good health.

Admittedly, it takes a little getting used to when making the switch to that many fresh fruits and vegetables. Start slowly. First, figure out what percentage of fruits and vegetables you are actually eating on a daily basis. Is it 5 percent, 25 percent, or closer to 50 percent of what you eat every day? Next, make a conscious effort to increase that percentage a little bit at a time. If you are accustomed to eating vegetables only with dinner, add some type of fresh vegetable to your lunch or midafternoon meal. I don't eat enough fresh fruit—so I experiment and try new or unusual fruits to keep it interesting! Ask at the produce counter what is especially new, good, or interesting.

Seasonal Eating

Adding fresh fruits and vegetables to your life is easier to adapt to if you learn to explore the wonderful seasonal produce in your grocery store or local farmer's market. Certain items will appear in abundance in your market during certain seasons. For instance, I find delicious fresh asparagus in the stores in May and June. July reminds me of peaches, peaches, peaches! In the fall months there is a wide and varied selection of different types of apples, and in the winter months there is an abundance of root vegetables. Seasonal shopping or seasonal eating is actually the very basis of macrobiotics, which has been around for centuries.

You will find that your body will respond swiftly and positively to seasonal eating. The chemistry makes perfect sense when you think about it. The coolness and high water volume of summer fruits such as watermelon and berries help to keep your body hydrated during the hot summer months when you need more liquids. The more dense, more carbohydrate-laden winter root vegetables such as potatoes, carrots, parsnips, celery root, and turnips work to store up energy in your body, thus keeping you warmer during the cold of winter. Seasonal foods also possess the specific vitamins and minerals necessary to keep your body functioning at its best during each season. Seasonal eating is commonsense eating. In the days before prepared food, eating with the seasons is how our ancestors survived—eating only what came out of the ground or off the trees season to season.

Do Not Deny Yourself Any Type of Food

There is no such thing as a good food or a bad food. Don't set up unrealistic laws to govern the food you eat, such as "I will never eat cookies again." Instead, make statements to yourself like "I will try all sorts of foods—not denying myself anything—and strive most of the time to eat those foods that make my body feel the best it possibly can." If you experiment and try different types of food, you will discover that some will make you feel better than others. So choosing what you want to *eat* is really choosing how you want to *feel*. Some foods will slow you down. Some will energize you. Some will fill you up. Others will leave you wanting more. It's up to you to choose *what* you want to eat and *how* you want to feel.

By denying yourself any type of food, say, for instance, chocolate, you only set yourself up for a total mind-and-body-absorbing chocolate obsession. And when you *do* finally "break down" and eat it after having been in a long, tortuous state of denial, you will likely overeat it. Deprivation leads to overindulgence. This is one of the main reasons that traditional dieting often backfires.

Instead, if it's chocolate you want, have a piece exactly when you want it. Taste it. Enjoy it. Allow it. Bless it. Celebrate the fact that you are eating *exactly* what you want, *exactly* when you want it. No longings, no cravings, no more deprivation.

Be Picky—Be Proud

You are special and unique with your own special and unique food needs. Don't settle for food that does not suit you or food that has been prepared in a way you do not like. Be choosy, be selective, insisting on *exactly* what makes your body feel best, as well as what is most pleasing and satisfying to your taste.

I became discriminating (or "picky") about my food when I recognized that in *every other* area of my life I am very selective. I am selective about my friends, my work, my doctors, my clothes, everything! When it came to food, however, I was *completely* indiscriminate. I would eat whatever I was served, or whatever was convenient or available—even if I didn't like it or if I really deep down wanted something else. By being decidedly nonselective about my food choices, I was attempting to call attention *away* from myself and what I chose to eat. In the process of all this I was never eating what I *really* desired and found myself eating "on the sly" to make up for it. My relationship with food changed for the better when I decided to become very selective.

Being a "picky" eater is not a bad thing. Being selective means you won't eat just *anything.* It implies that you are in touch with yourself and have a very clear picture of which foods keep your body functioning at its best and that you have the assertiveness and self-confidence to ask for what you want. I try to practice a healthy, polite selectivity about my food, especially when eating in restaurants where I don't have the same control as when I am in my own kitchen.

When dining out, I will consider the choices and then make the best choice from what's available. That choice will more than likely entail some special requests or slight alterations in how my order is prepared. I will ask for the fish to be baked with lemon only, or ask for sauce on the side. I like my vegetables steamed, so I usually ask for them to be prepared as such. If I don't like the type of bread being served, I ask for a different type. My friends and family always joke about how "high maintenance" I am when we are in a restaurant because it always takes me longer to order. I smile and say, "Thank you!" I *am* high maintenance and am proud of it. I know exactly what it takes to keep me looking and feeling terrific and I am confident enough to ask for it!

And not so surprisingly, I discovered that people are usually *more* than happy to accommodate your special food needs. Be sure you make your requests with a smile, and a "please" and you, too, will receive a favorable response *and* the food you want! Remember, you and your beautiful body deserve it!

Have food, will travel. If you are going somewhere where you know there will be food that is not your favorite, take your own food with you. I frequently make three- or four-hour car trips for business and pleasure. I always pack my favorite food to take along, as I generally don't like typical roadside fare. Be prepared and think ahead. Anticipate your food needs and take care of them in your *own* way and with the food *you* desire.

Being proud of the food you eat means no more hiding! For so many years I ate on the sly—eating when no one else was looking, sneaking food, popping a bite of some "forbidden" food in my mouth while I was in the kitchen. Sound familiar?

My relationship with food took a significant change for the better when I stopped being embarrassed and starting being proud of what I ate. Don't ever apologize or feel embarrassment about the food you choose to eat. Buy, order, cook, and eat your food with pride—knowing that it will work to nourish and satisfy your body in the best possible way.

Be Cool with Your Food

Being cool means learning to adapt a relaxed attitude about your food. No matter what, don't freak out over food—it will only spin you back into the negative diet, denial, guilt cycle all over again. Watch people who you think are "normal" eaters. They tend to stay calm about food in spite of the circumstances. They maintain a sense of ease and relaxed confidence no matter what food situation they are faced with.

Strive to maintain your own state of normal eating. "Normal" will be slightly different for everyone. Normal eating means that sometimes you eat a little too much and sometimes you don't eat quite enough—yet neither of these extremes throws you off balance. Balance is the key.

Picture eating like riding a bicycle. If you are riding with your body tensed up—very rigid and inflexible—when you hit a bump in the road (and you will), you will likely fall off and get hurt. But if you ride *calmly* with a *relaxed, flexible* motion, when you hit a bump you will move *through* the bump, without being thrown off by it. When you are loose and relaxed you absorb the bumps.

Keep calm, smooth, and flexible with your food so that when the bumps come, you are able to move right through them with the minimum of agitation, stress, or displacement.

What I've Learned about My Food Needs

Many women I work with ask me what I eat and what works for me. The first thing I tell them is that what *I* do might not be right for them. No two bodies will relate to food or eating patterns in the same way. However, through many years of trial and error and a die-hard determination to discover ways to eat harmoniously with my body, I will share with you exactly how I strive to relate to food.

It is important that you notice I use the word *strive.* Strive means that some days are better than others. Strive means that I have accepted the fact that food and I will have an ever-evolving relationship—with no two days being alike. So, what do I do? I try to follow the guidelines I have just given in the previous pages and I keep a few key concepts in mind that I have found to be useful for my body. Maybe they will be useful for you too. Use what you can, forget the rest. But please check with your doctor before you significantly change any of your eating habits.

I strive daily to maintain what I call a state of food homeostasis—meaning, I try never to find myself being either too hungry or too full. If I am too hungry (starving) it means that I have waited too long to answer my body's signal to eat and I will generally overeat as a result. If I am too full, it means I *definitely* waited too long to eat, and have overeaten, thus further muting my body's signaling devices.

To achieve my food homeostasis balance, I try to eat five or six *smaller* meals a day instead of three larger "square" meals. My body responds best if I have a little something to eat every three to four hours. I find that maintaining this balance stabilizes my metabolism and keeps my energy at a near-constant "peak" level throughout the day.

Many women respond well to multiple, small "feedings" as opposed to a few big meals. In fact, some theories suggest that the three-meals-a-day ritual is outdated. A nutritionist once told me that eating only three times a day was a practice popularized during the Industrial Revolution when factory owners were trying to achieve maximum worker output with minimum scheduled feeding times. And that, in fact, our bodies perform optimally when fed small amounts every few hours. Try it for a day or two and see how you feel.

My body also needs some sort of protein before noon. If I don't eat protein with my first "meal" of the day, I will be *sure* to have some sort of meat, fish, eggs, or cheese around noontime. If I eat just a bit of protein early on, I have more energy and fewer cravings.

I *do* strive to watch my fat intake—however, I don't keep a check on this for "weight" reasons but rather for how my body *feels.* If I eat an excess of fats or oils, my body feels sluggish and slow. If I stick to mostly fruits, vegetables, and carbohydrates, I wake up feeling better each morning. And that's the bottom line, right? How we feel when we open our eyes each day usually has an impact on how we will feel throughout the rest of the day.

I drink mostly water, juices, and tea. I drink very little alcohol because it makes my body feel bloated and puffy. I've asked around and many nutritionists and doctors believe that water is still the perfect drink for satisfying thirst and cleansing the body. Think of your body as a washing machine and your insides as the clothes you want to wash. If you want the clothes to get clean, you wash them with water, not diet soda, right?

And finally, I bless my food silently before I eat. By blessing I mean that I take a moment to thank my food for the work it is going to perform within my body. I further ask it to please metabolize and burn in the most useful and effective way possible for my body. By taking just a few seconds to think about these things, I find that I much more consciously enjoy what I eat.

Our negative feelings associated with food *can* change over time if we adopt a relaxed, rational attitude about our food. Remain calm about eating. Make sure you are asking for and receiving the type of food you truly want, and then enjoy it! Breaking bread with family and friends is one of the great pleasures of life. Don't allow old thought patterns and preconceived notions to affect that pleasure.

In my mind, the complement to inputting food is outputting energy, or movement, which we will now explore further in Step 8.

1. "I [*insert name*] promise never to "diet" again. I hereby release my body and mind from the endless cycle of deprivation and guilt. Instead I will try to make peace with my food while listening to and being guided by my body's natural intelligence."

2. Figure out what percentage of fresh fruits and vegetables you are currently eating every day. Think of ways to increase that percentage little by little.

3. Discover your local farmer's market or fresh produce stand. Talk to the farmer or your local greengrocer and ask questions about which fruits and vegetables are in season.

4. Make a list of your ten favorite foods.

_____   _____
_____   _____
_____   _____
_____   _____
_____   _____

Acknowledge that these foods are neither good nor bad. Allow yourself to enjoy your favorite foods when and where you please, without guilt or hiding.

5. Whenever you are eating in a restaurant, practice "picky eating." Order your food prepared exactly how you desire. Practice an air of polite assertiveness, being very descriptive about your food needs and desires.

6. Make a practice of silently blessing your food before you eat it. Ask your body to metabolize and convert the food to energy in the most efficient way. Visualize in your mind how well the food is nourishing your body and how wonderful it will make you feel.

*A*foot
and light-hearted
I take to the
open road,
Healthy, free,
the world
before me. . . .

—WALT WHITMAN

8

Explore Options in Movement

I use the word "movement" because moving is so much more than "exercising" or "working out." Movement is everything you do involving your body. Moving is raking leaves, walking to the car, climbing the stairs, dancing around the living room, and picking up your children. Movement also includes running a marathon or taking an aerobics class, but it is not limited to these activities. Movement is *all-encompassing,* whereas exercise can be limited.

The word "exercise" makes me think it is going to hurt . . . movement just sounds like something I would rather do. Exercise evokes images of ungraceful machines with intimidating names—butt-masters, thigh-masters, stair machines, and ab-gadgets. Movement makes me think of dancers and beautiful, slow, fluid motions. Essentially, it boils down to the simple fact that I can comfortably commit to "moving" for the rest of my life—something I cannot say about exercise.

Exercise is a subset of movement. The word "exercise" holds the connotation of a stern regimen, of weight loss and guilt. To me, exercise carries the implication that we are having to fix something that is "wrong," "out of shape," or "bad." Movement isn't about fixing anything at all. Instead, it is a celebration of all that is *right* with our bodies.

Moving makes you feel alive. It boosts your energy level and improves your mood. Movement makes you *stronger and longer*—but more on that later. I have yet to meet anyone who hasn't reaped endless benefits—both emotional and physical—by increasing their movement.

All for Moving . . . Movement for All!

Movement isn't an exclusive club that we are unable to join. As well-rounded women, we are entitled to every option and variation of movement. We do not have to wait to begin moving. We do not need anyone's permission to allow us to move. (Although I do *strongly* advise that you let your doctor know if you decide to intensify or increase your movement.) Movement is not size discriminatory. It is open, unlimited, and for all of us to enjoy.

Movement does not begin when we wear a certain size, weigh a magic number, or achieve a certain level of "fitness." It is not limited to time or place when we perceive we will be thinner, lighter, skinnier, or in better shape. I often hear that excuse from the women I work with. They say they will begin moving when they are in better shape. "Better shape" comes from moving, not tomorrow, but today.

Movement is adaptable to our own individual needs and on our own terms. It's a highly personal choice of when, where, and how you choose to move. You might want to dance or walk or stretch. Maybe you want to take a swim or a hike or play a game of tennis. How you move today does not have to resemble in any way how you moved in the past or how you plan to move in the future.

Movement is not a punishment for being large. Rather, it is a gift you give to yourself at any size. Before you are ready to receive this gift, however, you might need to clear out some old misconceptions and negative thought patterns about movement.

The Ghost of PE Classes Past

Gym class almost killed the concept of movement for me. I was a fat kid and I hated phys ed. It was a routine, both painful and embarrassing, and one from which I couldn't escape for most of my childhood and teen years. Gym class treats all kids the same—even though we are not. In school, there is no consideration of our shape, our size, our natural abilities or proclivities, our interest level or our desire. PE, for a child in school, is everything that movement as an adult is *not*.

Gym class brought out my worst insecurities. Will I have to weigh in? Will the assigned gym suits fit me? Will I have to take a shower in the "gang" showers? Will I get picked for a team? Will I be chosen *last* as always? Can I make it around the track? Will we have to do the President's Fitness Council test again this year? (Asking me to hold a chin-up for thirty seconds when I cannot hold it for even one.) It's no wonder that PE turned me against every physical activity or movement.

So, let me state for the record—this is not your sixth grade gym class. There is no attendance being taken. You will not be weighed. There are no mandatory chin-ups. You can wear whatever you want. There are no teams or sides. You can move at your own pace, not the pace the President's Fitness Council dictates. You are safe. I promise. And you are going to find that you enjoy moving on your own terms and in the ways that are most comfortable for your own body.

Release the Future . . . Enjoy the Now

As a culture, we have become completely misguided in our motivation for moving. Try asking any health-club junkie *why* they are doing what they are doing. I'll bet they say something akin to "to lose weight," "to pump up," "to get a better body," "to get abs of steel," "to look better in a bathing suit," and on and on and on. But, how many people do you think will answer, "Because I like the way it makes my body feel today"?

In order to make movement a permanent part of our daily lives, we need to release the idea that we are moving only to achieve some *future* goal or state of *future* fitness. Movement becomes joyous when you concentrate on the *here* and *now*—how your body will feel today—not six months from now. Change your focus from a future *look* to a right-this-minute *feeling*.

Work to become more in touch with how you feel when you move. Are you feeling alive? Exhilarated? Happy? Maybe even tired? Content? Is your heart pumping fast? Do you feel heated up? Does your body "kick in" at a certain point? And, after you move, does a feeling of well-being set in? Does your skin look better because your blood has been vigorously circulated, creating a healthy glow? Does your mind feel more clear and focused? Do you sit up straighter?

These are all feelings you can experience from paying attention to the here and now. If you are focusing only on the future you will miss the joyous moments that will make you want to move every day. And here's the secret. All of those future looks and future fitness goals will take care of themselves over time if you are moving solely for the joy of it today.

Types of Movement

There are two types of movement that I am going to differentiate between. *Functional* movement is every type of moving that we do as we progress through our daily lives—at work, at home, doing any activity, errand, chore, or duty that we normally have to perform day to day. *Recreational* movement, on the other hand, is anything that you *plan ahead* to do, *make time* to do or, *dress appropriately* to do outside of your daily responsibilities or regimen. The thing to remember here is that *both* types count as movement—one is not better or worse than the other; they are just different.

For those just beginning a commitment to movement, it is advisable to start by increasing or intensifying your daily *functional* movements. Climb the stairs instead of taking the escalator. Walk to the corner drugstore instead of driving there. Rake the leaves yourself instead of paying the neighborhood kids to do it. Seek a parking space farther away from where you are going instead of closer, and walk the extra four or five rows. Simply put, a few minor changes in the way you move through your daily life routines (functional movements) can significantly increase your overall movement level.

Recreational movements are movements you choose to make time to do outside of your daily functional routine and include exercise class, fitness training, dance, and all sports. Recreational movement can be a stretch class at the health club, a half-hour-a-day swim at the YWCA pool, a brisk walk on the treadmill, or a game of tennis on a Saturday afternoon. Golf, aerobics, weight training in the gym, swimming laps, race walking, skiing, rowing, and yoga are all examples of recreational movement. *Recreational* movement is the focus of this step.

Different Bodies, Different Needs

Everyone's movement needs are different. I can't endorse one form of recreational movement over another, since all of our bodies are so completely different. In fact, I am surprised when I see someone on television, in a video, or in the magazines telling me the "best" way to move. How can they possibly know that? They do not know me, my body, my lifestyle, my likes, or dislikes.

Many women I talk to feel the same although they may not be able to put a reason to the feeling. Exercise "plans," fitness "routines," workout "regimens," and all those gadgets are created for the masses, not individual bodies. Be wary of their claims that their way is the *only* way, or the *best* method. If you listen to or read an advertisement for a specific movement "tool," you can bet that they will be saying things like "Get back into shape," "Lose weight," "Firm up," "Summer is coming," and other assorted exercise-by-intimidation statements.

Try not to fall for such scare tactics. Each of our bodies is unique and we are learning to move for *the joy of moving as we are experiencing it today* rather than anticipating future "washboard abs" or dramatic, life-altering weight loss. If you *do* discover a way of moving that you enjoy and that uses a tape or a gadget, go right ahead and use it with your newfound wisdom about movement. Add it to the mix of your personal movement options and enjoy it for the way it makes you feel today!

There is no single type of movement that is correct for everyone. We are all so different in our movement needs that instead of talking about specific *types* of movement, I want to share with you a *philosophy* of moving. This philosophy will provide a *framework* into which every woman can fit her own specific movements and activities. I call this framework Strong and Long.

Strong and Long

Strong and Long is my way of describing and categorizing the yin and yang of all movement. Strong and Long work hand in hand as an interdependent duality within our bodies. It is a framework within which everyone can build and explore movement. The goal is to be both Strong and Long, and yet each is achieved in a slightly different way. Allow me to explain further.

The concept of Strong and Long is based on the idea that for every *movement* there is a *countermovement*. For every *crunch,* there is a *stretch*. For every *compression,* there is an *elongation*. For every *flex,* there is a *point*. Different movements are primarily geared to making your body either Stronger or Longer. Some do both. Strong and Long are married. They go hand in hand.

Ballet dancers and swimmers are my inspiration for Strong and Long. Dancing and swimming are ways of moving that create strong, elongated bodies—bodies that are simultaneously tight and fluid, strong and flexible. As a well-rounded woman, I look at strong, long dancers' or swimmers' bodies and strive to incorporate *some* of their qualities and characteristics into my own. This does *not* mean that I attempt to look exactly as they do. I take the attributes I admire and work to translate them in a manner that is appropriate for my own body. We'll start with Strong.

Why Be Strong?

Strong is one half of this effective combination. But what does it mean to be strong? Being strong means different things to different people. We all have our personal strong goals. Strong involves both *strength* (sheer muscle power) and *endurance* (cardiovascular capability).

For me being strong means that I can climb the stairs in my house without huffing and puffing; that I can run after (and catch) my cat if she escapes out of the house; that I can help my neighbor carry her groceries from her car to the house with ease; that I am able to move my furniture around my house whenever I get in the mood to redecorate; that I can carry in big armloads of firewood from the garage. I enjoy being strong enough to play two or three sets of tennis without feeling like I am going to collapse; strong so I can take long, invigorating walks in the countryside; as well as being strong enough to rotate and flip my bed mattress by myself when necessary. Think about the different types of strong goals you might have for your own life.

In order to become strong you need to participate in movements that will work to increase both your strength and your endurance. Getting stronger includes most aerobic and cardiovascular activities—in other words, any movement that will increase and sustain your heart rate for a period of time. Strong also incorporates some anaerobic activities such as weight (or resistance) training. The following is a partial list of movements and activities that can make you strong.

Aerobics classes of all types—high-impact, low-impact, step, slide, funk, cardio, circuit training, and body sculpting
Swimming (also makes you long)
Cycling
Walking/Hiking/Running
Cross-Country Skiing (also makes you long)
"Aerobic Machine" Training—i.e., treadmill, Stairmaster, Nordic track
Rowing—canoeing, kayaking, etc.

Jump Rope
In-line Skating—better known as Roller Blading
Weight Training (also called resistance training)— although technically nonaerobic (anaerobic), using machine weights or free weights increases lean muscle mass and overall strength.

There are endless ways and means of getting strong. Team sports, if played regularly, can make you strong. Dance class such as jazz or modern can also work to make you strong. Try different strong activities, noticing which ones fit comfortably and easily into your lifestyle. Strong is one half of the combination. Strong's faithful counterpart is Long.

Why Be Long?

Long is the second half of my two-part movement philosophy. Long is exactly what it sounds like. Getting longer involves those movements and/or activities that work to make your body stretch, elongate, and lengthen. Long is not a new concept. Watch any professional athlete before a competition. They always take time to stretch— allowing their muscles to get longer—before they begin their sport, whether it be football, marathon running, or figure skating.

I recognized the importance of getting long by watching women (and men) during the exercise-intense 1980s. Here's what I saw over the course of the years. As these women were *overdoing* it in gyms and health clubs around the country—striving for the perfect, worked-out body (whatever *that* is!) they were focusing on strong without the long. I would watch in amazement as they would sometimes take two or even three aerobics classes a day and then spend an hour lifting weights. They believed that the more crunches, the more high kicks, the more push-ups, and the more jumping jacks they did, the closer they would get to the "body of their dreams." They spent most of their time getting *strong,* to use our new term, but what they were forgetting to do was to get *long* by stretching and elongating the muscles they had just been overworking.

As a result, I noticed a trend of "gym bodies" that certainly looked lean, but more than that, appeared "crunched up," "squatty," "compressed," and downright bulky in some cases. These women had ignored the importance of *stretch* (long), because they thought if it didn't make them hurt, sweat, or frenetically burn calories, it wasn't worth doing.

It was from my observations of these women that I knew strong *had* to be accompanied by long or else we would all end up with those stubby little worked-out bodies. Once I recognized the duality and the interdependence of the two, it began to make more and more sense to me. Yin and Yang. Day and Night. Black and White. Strong and Long.

Like strong, there are countless ways of getting long. Getting long is about *stretching* your body. Stretching can be done anytime and anywhere. Most simply, you can stretch by lying on the floor flat on your back and reaching your arms over your head as far as they will reach while pointing and stretching your legs straight out at the same time. This simple stretch is a great way to elongate your body first thing in the morning or anytime you have been confined to one position for a long period of time. You can also do a simple stretch when you are seated by making a conscious effort to sit up perfectly straight, relaxing your shoulders but holding your spine straight and tall while imagining that you are creating space between

242

each of the vertebrae along your back. These are two of the most simple ways through which you can make stretching a part of your daily routine.

You can also work on getting longer by participating in a stretch class. Most health clubs as well as the YWCA offer a selection of stretch classes. Usually about an hour in length, the classes will take you through a head-to-toe stretch, working and elongating every part of your body. Other long options to consider:

Yoga is an excellent way to stretch your body and a wonderful form of movement for women of size. Yoga makes me long, improves my flexibility, regulates my breathing, increases blood circulation, and gives me an all-over healthy feeling of well-being. There are many types of yoga to explore but all yoga is centered around breathing and stretching. Through the practice of yoga one discovers an *internal* furnace and learns to fuel it with controlled breathing.

Yoga movements are made slowly and internally. With a bit of research you will find specialized yoga studios as well as yoga classes being taught at health clubs and exercise studios around the country. If you would prefer trying yoga in your home, there are a variety of videotapes available that will guide you through the different yoga positions and philosophy. (See Resources.)

Callanetics is a trademarked nonimpact movement plan involving a series of deep-muscular contracting and stretching movements (in "triple slow-motion"), which work to elongate the muscles. Callanetics is very woman-of-size friendly. There is no special equipment required and it offers a variety of ways to participate with Callanetics books and videotapes as well as approximately twenty licensed Callanetics studios across the country where you can take a Callanetics class.

Pilates is a seventy-five-year-old, nonimpact method of movement that strengthens, elongates, and tones the muscles. Popular among dancers and in its purest form, Pilates is done in a one-on-one session with an instructor and using *specific* equipment that works to strengthen muscles while elongating them at the same time. There is special emphasis on "correcting" individual body needs while strengthening the "core"—the midsection of the body from which all movement effectively stems. These days, there are Pilates-inspired classes springing up in health clubs around the country. These classes incorporate the Pilates philosophy of stretching and elongating through light resistance and slow repetition within a general "stretch and tone" class.

The Alexander Technique was created by F. M. Alexander, an Australian actor and reciter at the turn of the century, as he was attempting to correct a voice problem he was having. What he discovered was that the misalignment of his body (stemming from his spine, naturally) was causing the problem, and with proper alignment he not only fixed his voice but improved his general health as well.

The Alexander Technique is a process of aligning and straightening the spine with the guidance and direction of a certified Alexander teacher. In addition to improving one's posture and giving the sensation of being *stretched,* Alexander work can improve performance in many activities, including walking and sitting, as well as most athletic activities. After just a few Alexander sessions, I noticed that I was performing every movement of my life in a new way—conscious and aware of the *length* of my body, walking and moving more gracefully and with a sense of elongation.

As you work on becoming long, you create "space" between the vertebrae and can actually appear *taller.*

Your back will strengthen and stretch, supporting you upwards and creating an elongated, more vertical appearance. As you begin to practice being long, you will notice immediate differences in how you look and feel. Your clothes will fit differently because creating length allows clothes to hang, not cling. Becoming long is a positive way of truly embracing all the space you occupy. Stretch and elongate into every last inch of it!

The Back-Belly Connection

More so than any other area of the body, your "core"— the area around your midsection including the lower belly and lower back—is the location from which most movement stems. The strength of this core is contingent upon the strong, symbiotic relationship between the lower back and the lower belly.

The lower portion of the body—our core—is the base from which we center and carry the rest of our weight. Living in an ample body, I can attest to the fact that this is a crucial area to keep strong and healthy. As well-rounded women, we are more prone to experience lower back pain and distress, because we carry more weight. This distress can take many forms, including general lower back pain, difficulty lying flat on our backs (without bending the knees), or even difficulty getting up comfortably from low seating.

All of these conditions arise from a weak central core. Several years ago I was fortunate enough to come into contact with a sports medicine specialist who enlightened me about the simple yet insightful connection between the belly and the back. Keeping strong lower belly muscles helps to support the lower back and vice versa, which together create a stronger core. The goal here is *not* washboard abs or flat stomachs. The goal is inner strength of the lower belly, flexibility and strength of the lower back, and a solid core to enable us to better support and carry our weight.

Try utilizing this way of thinking when considering abdominal or lower body (core) movements—thinking not of flattening the stomach, but rather of *strengthening the core*.

The Privilege of Movement

Take a moment to recognize what an extreme privilege it is to be moving your body in the ways you choose. So many cannot because of injury or illness. Celebrate the ways, means, and locales of your movements. Celebrate the scenery, the nature, and the sights. Revel like a child just released from class for recess. Take deep breaths of fresh air. Allow movement to be a special gift you give to your body every day.

I really started to notice how privileged I was to be able to move and take in the world around me one day several years ago when I was taking my "power" walk in New York City's Central Park. It was a beautiful, cold, crisp day and from where I was doing my walking I could enjoy a panoramic view of Manhattan's incredible skyline. It felt as if I were in the middle of a jewelry box with all of the shining buildings like rare jewels around me.

A few moments before I had been getting a little weary, but once I really saw and took in the beauty of the day and of my surroundings I discovered newfound energy within me. I picked up my walk to a nice even jog and in my mind dedicated the whole beautiful outing to those who cannot move as they wish. It *is* a privilege to be able to move.

Useful Tips for Better Movement Experiences

1. Use the right clothing and gear. It will make all the difference in the world. Most importantly, *insist* on owning shoes that will give you the support you need for your movement choices. Your best bet is to purchase shoes at an athletic footwear specialty store; they will have the best selection and be able to better serve your special needs.

Choose clothes or "active wear" that fit loosely and comfortably, that will encourage breathability and freedom of movement. There are several very good mail-order resources for large-size active wear. (See Resources). In addition, many department stores have active-wear departments that carry women's workout gear up to size 3X. I have also discovered that the Eddie Bauer catalogue (See Resources) carries active wear, both inner wear as well as outer gear, up to women's size XXL (20–22) and up to XXXL in men's sizes.

If your movement involves other "gear," ask lots of questions before you buy. Seek out knowledgeable salespeople who will be able to address your specific movement and/or sports needs. Be bold. Be educated. Ask for what you want and need.

2. Don't plan your movement too far in advance. If you do, you run the risk of ignoring your body's signals of what type of movement it needs on a particular day. I find that women who set a rigid course for themselves rarely stick to a long-term, lifetime commitment to moving.

Movement should reflect what your body feels like doing on any given day. Granted, we *do* have to push a little to get ourselves up and moving, but by and large the body will let you know what type of movement it needs to do. I "hear" very clearly the days when my body craves a "get strong" movement such as a brisk walk, a sweaty "funk" class, or an hour of weight training and resistance at the health club. Other days, my body will cry to "get long"—meaning I will take a yoga class or perhaps just spend a half hour on the living room floor stretching. Once you start to "listen," your body *will* let you know *exactly* how it wants to move.

Europeans are so much more advanced than we are when it comes to movement—allowing their *environment* and their *mood* to influence their movement options. Generally speaking, they are less obsessed with the body and the fanatic "workout" mentality that pervades America. When I asked my Austrian friend how he keeps "in shape," he looked at me incredulously and said, "I don't *try* to keep in shape. I ski and skate in the winter because there is the snow and the mountain; and, in the warmer months I go on long hikes and picnic lunches because the weather is so nice." Now isn't that a heck of a lot more civilized than thrashing our bodies around on a Stairmaster to the point of exhaustion?!

3. Find your movement "groove." This is easier to *feel* than to explain. You'll know what I mean once you feel it for the first time. When you begin to explore movement on a regular basis, you will experience many new sensations within your body. Your "groove" is that specific range of motion (usually very small at first) for any movement you do, wherein your body tells you that you are working at the right rhythm, the right speed, and the right intensity.

You will be able to identify this groove by a realization that your body is performing a specific movement with effective ease. You will feel your muscles *engaged* and *strong*, and a natural rhythm, gait, or flow will ensue. You will find your groove in every movement you do. There is a groove you will hit when you are walking, swimming, dancing, or stretching.

In tennis, when the ball connects with the racquet at the optimal place on the face of the racquet, it is called the "sweet spot." That is the point where everything connects and engages to achieve maximum performance or the best shot. Your *groove* is like your sweet spot. It is the feeling of moving at an optimal level of performance for your body for that particular time and day. Grooves can change. It might be easier to find your groove on certain days and not on others. It's always there. Strive to find it and allow it to guide your safe and effective execution of the movement.

4. Approach fitness clubs/gyms with caution and information. Are you considering joining a health club or gym? A club is a wonderful environment to enjoy any number of movement options, all under one roof. I am a member of a health club because it offers a wide variety of classes ranging from yoga to boxing. I also enjoy some of their amenities such as the steam room and sauna. The key to finding the gym of your choice is to know *in advance* exactly what you are looking for.

Generally speaking, health clubs are for those who like to participate in movements *with* other people. In a club environment you are going to come into contact with many people. It can be a substantially different experience from moving alone, so you should know what you are used to doing or prefer doing. Would you be joining a club to take classes or just to use the equipment? Do you care about the extras such as sauna, steam, massage, etc.? Are you interested in the option of one-on-one training, and is that available? Would you feel more comfortable in a club just for women? Find out about the instructors and/or fitness professionals who run the club. What are their backgrounds? Do any have experience with women (or men) of size? Can they accommodate your special needs and requests? These are the types of questions you will want to ask before you decide to join a club.

Ask for a day pass or a couple of free class passes from the club you are interested in joining. By actually participating in the activities, if only for an hour, you will get a much better idea of the feel of the club. And, remember, proximity is *everything*. You will be 100 percent more likely to commit to movement in your new club if it's not a hassle to get there. If you want to go there directly after work, choose a club near the office. My health club is a five-minute walk from my house. I love the flexibility of being able to decide on the spur of the moment and then *go*! The closer it is and the easier it is to get to, the more likely you are to honor a commitment to moving there! A final word of advice. Avoid "lifetime" memberships to anything.

5. Flex your options. Try everything. Keep folding in new ways of moving to the old mix. Keep it fresh to keep it interesting. If you swim, alternate it with a day of walking. If you walk, try an evening yoga class. Skip, jump, box, sprint, stretch. Try it all. See what you like and find out how many different ways you can move your body.

I find I go through stages. I will spend several months where all I want to do is go for long "power walks" listening to books on tape in my headset. Then I will do a complete 180-degree turn and launch into weeks of box-aerobics class at my health club. By changing things whenever I feel like it, I keep my commitment to movement fresh and interesting. It's okay to change things a little. In fact, if you *do* make a habit of exploring all types of movement, you'll constantly be finding new things you enjoy doing. Don't limit yourself to the same class, routine, or route day in and day out. Mixing it up means you'll keep it up!

6. Rest. All professional athletes know the value of allowing the body a chance to rest and rejuvenate. Just as your body is a perfect machine and will let you know when it wants to eat or move, it, too, will tell you in no uncertain terms when it needs to rest. I usually give myself one day of rest for every three days of movement—but this ratio will be different for everyone.

In order to maintain a commitment to moving and working toward a longer, stronger body, you have to rest. Resting gives the body a chance to catch up, regroup, and assimilate all the long and/or strong movements you have been doing. If you don't allow the body proper time to rest, all the wonderful benefits of movement can be lost. Your performance level, intensity, and urge to move regularly will increase if you allow ample rest time.

7. Check it out with your doctor. Be safe and check out any new movement plans with your doctor. Let them know exactly what you are going to be doing. Any good doctor with whom you have an open relationship should be supportive and might even offer suggestions or ask you to update them on a regular basis.

Movement is a privilege and a gift. Enjoy the movement you are able to do each day. Make it part of the new, well-rounded you!

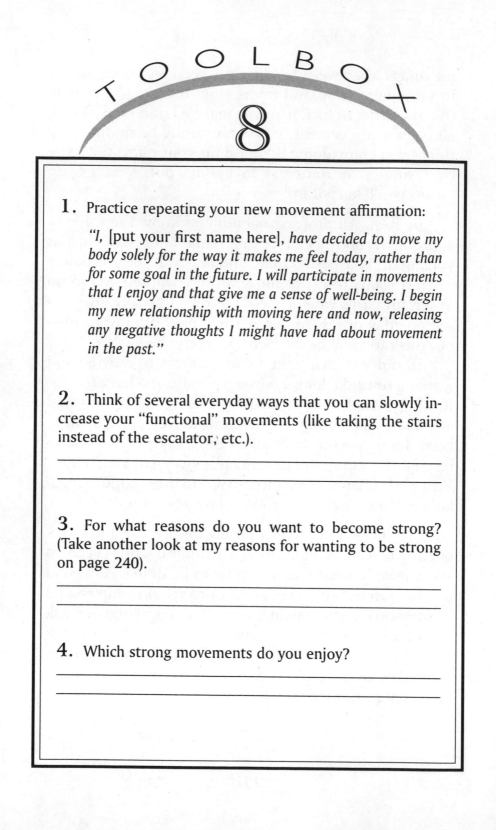

TOOLBOX 8

1. Practice repeating your new movement affirmation:

"I, [put your first name here], have decided to move my body solely for the way it makes me feel today, rather than for some goal in the future. I will participate in movements that I enjoy and that give me a sense of well-being. I begin my new relationship with moving here and now, releasing any negative thoughts I might have had about movement in the past."

2. Think of several everyday ways that you can slowly increase your "functional" movements (like taking the stairs instead of the escalator, etc.).

_____

_____

3. For what reasons do you want to become strong? (Take another look at my reasons for wanting to be strong on page 240).

_____

_____

4. Which strong movements do you enjoy?

_____

_____

5. Think of a few reasons that long will be good for your own body. Posture? Alignment? Standing taller? Alleviating back pain? Stretching out from work requirements (either from sitting too long or strenuous physical work)?

_____

_____

6. What are some ways to become long that you would enjoy?

_____

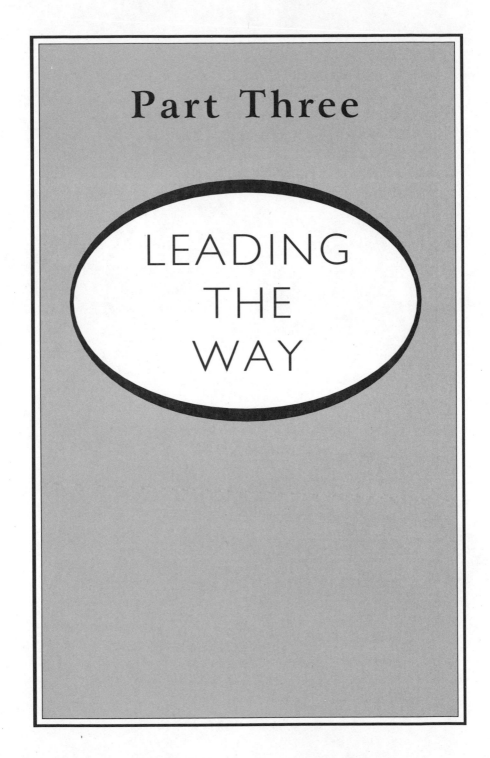

Part Three

LEADING THE WAY

*C*ongratulations. You have now completed the eight steps and are on your way to becoming a new, confident, well-rounded you! Let's take a quick look at how far you have come.

- You have learned to balance your expectations and old thought patterns dealing with your body and now believe in the power you have to change your own life.
- You now know the importance of making the crucial time you need to relax, and how to use simple daily meditations to keep yourself centered, productive, and happy.
- You have initiated a new relationship with your body, working to mend any wounds from past breakups. You have taken inventory of your inner strengths— learning that you are much, much more than just your body.
- You have armed yourself with a head-to-toe outer assessment—rediscovering and celebrating all your positive assets.
- You now know the fashion industry's well-kept secret of systematic dressing and can now uncover your own personal uniform and enjoy getting dressed with ease and confidence.
- You know how to proportion your accessories (fashion *and* life accessories!) to fit your body and your needs.
- You began the ongoing and lifelong process of evaluating your relationship with food—working toward harmonious, peaceful respect for the food you eat.

- And you have started to explore the many options and ways you can move your body—moving for the joy of movement rather than for some nebulous future goal.

I hope you will continue to work through the steps, turning to them whenever you need to for guidance and support. They are my gift to you. Now, I want to enlist your help. I have a mission.

I believe that we, as well-rounded women, have the potential to be the leaders in a new body-acceptance movement—teaching women of all shapes and sizes how to gracefully and lovingly live inside the bodies they have. Who else is better for the job? If we are able to love and accept our own bodies as they are, we are in a position of strength to share our self-love with others. We have watched as today's society and its unrealistic body images have turned otherwise naturally healthy women into weight-obsessed, ill-nutritioned, overexercised neurotics, constantly searching for a state of "perfection" that does not exist. The more of us that stand up and say, "I don't buy it," the more we can begin to shape a world where women are united through a healthy bond of body acceptance, rather than body hatred.

We will be the women who love and accept ourselves and have love and acceptance to spare—ready and willing to share it with others. We will follow a regimen of physical, emotional, and spiritual health, accepting our bodies as they are—with all their strengths as well as their limitations. By learning to love our own bodies as they are, we are setting a new kind of example for others to follow. We will teach women how to love their own bodies in a nondestructive, realistic, and supportive way—acting as their guides on the journey to self acceptance.

Will you help by loving the well-rounded *you* first, and then share the message with others?

Resources

STEP 5: CREATE A UNIFORM

Bali's Lace N' Smooth all-in-one. Call Bali at 1-800-BALI-USA for store locations or mail orders.

J.C. Penney all-in-one available through J.C. Penney Catalog. Call 1-800-222-6161.

Great selection of foundation garments through Just My Size catalog. Call 1-800-IT FITS ME.

For more daring lingerie and undergarments, Fredericks of Hollywood now offers plus sizes! Call 1-800-323-9525 for a catalog.

Danskin legging shorts. Call 1-800-288-6749 for stores near you.

Margie Bags for clear accessory bags. Bags are $4.75 each. To order call 1-503-245-5352 or fax at 1-503-293-9440.

STEP 6: ACCESSORIZE YOUR LIFE APPROPRIATELY

Kenneth Jay Lane Jewelry. Call 1-800-552-0699 to order "Barbara Bush" pearls. Ask about custom sizes.

Jewelry "extenders" available through Robin Barr Enterprises. For order form, call 1-310-358-7351.

Resources

STEP 7: EVALUATE YOUR RELATIONSHIP WITH FOOD

SUGGESTED BOOKS OF INTEREST ON EATING AND FOOD

Chopra, Deepak. *Perfect Weight.* Harmony Books, 1994.

Fisher, M.K.F. *The Art of Eating.* Collier Books, 1990.

Haas, Elson M. *A Diet for All Seasons.* Celestial Arts, 1995.

Haas, Elson M. *Staying Healthy With the Seasons.* Celestial Arts, 1981.

Pitchfor, Paul. *Healing With Whole Foods.* North Atlantic Books, 1993.

STEP 8: EXPLORE OPTIONS IN MOVEMENT

CLOTHING AND GEAR

Beautiful Skier. Ski wear in plus sizes. Call 1-800-638-3334.

Dover Saddlery. Carries plus-size riding pants in black or beige for up to a forty-four-inch waist. Call 1-800-989-1500.

Eddie Bauer. Call 1-800-426-8020 for catalog.

Greater Salt Lake Clothing Company. Skiwear in larger sizes. Call 1-801-273-8700 for catalog.

Hot Off the Tour. Golf wear up to size 22. Call 1-800-944-8688.

Junonia. Exercise and active wear for larger sizes. Call 1-800-JUNONIA for catalog.

Water Wear. Swim wear up to size 28. Call 1-800-321-7848.

MOVEMENT TECHNIQUES/INFORMATION AND VIDEO

The Alexander Technique. For more information, look under "Alexander Technique" in phone book.

Callanetics. Call 1-800-8-CALLAN for more information and location of Callanetics studios around the country.

The Pilates Institute. For information on Pilates in your area call 1-505-988-1990.

Yoga for Round Bodies. Two-part yoga video series made just for women of size. To order, call 1-800-793-0666.